To my parents, for cheering me as I ran my own race

A RACE LIKE NO OTHER

26.2 Miles
Through the Streets of New York

LIZ ROBBINS

HARPER

An Imprint of HarperCollins*Publishers*
www.harpercollins.com

HarperCollins books may be purchased for educational, business, or sales promotional use. For information, please write: Special Markets Department, HarperCollins Publishers, 10 East 53rd Street, New York, NY 10022.

FIRST EDITION

Designed by Kara Strubel

Library of Congress Cataloging-in-Publication Data is available upon request.

ISBN: 978-0-06-137313-8

08 09 10 11 12   ID/RRD   10 9 8 7 6 5 4 3 2 1

CONTENTS

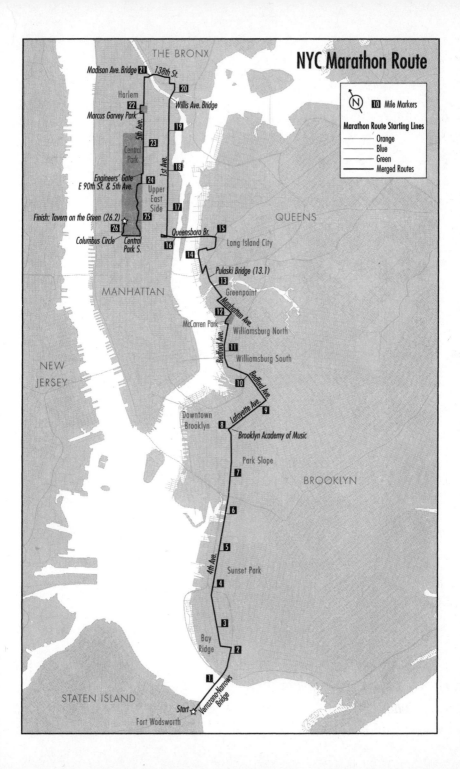

A RACE LIKE NO OTHER

INTRODUCTION

Marathoners push themselves to the edge of insanity and exhaustion, because when they look back on those 26.2 miles, the view is profoundly satisfying.

They see where they have been and what they have become.

Distance running is a pastime uniquely suited to introspection. To run is to question why. To run the New York City Marathon is to discover the answer.

A total of 749,791 people have crossed the finish line in Central Park since the first New York City Marathon in 1970. They all have a reason why they participate in the race, whether they run to live or they live to run.

They run with mothers and fathers, with brothers and sisters, with husbands and wives, or they run with their memories.

They come to outrun their demons and their diagnoses.

They run with members of a team, sometimes tethered to a blind runner by a shoestring.

They race on wheels if they cannot run.

They run to check it off the life list.

They run to eat cake or to chase vanity.

They run to suffer so others will not.

They run because they cannot stop running.

They run to win.

And at the end of the day, at the end of five bridges and five boroughs and 26.2 miles, they will have run because it is New York and they are not alone.

On Sunday, November 4, 2007, some 39,265 participants swarmed the Verrazano-Narrows Bridge, making New York's the largest marathon in the world for the fourth year in a row.

Like so much in this city of eight million people, the race is all about volume. Not just in numbers, but decibels. Two million fans, an unscientific estimate by city officials, stand and shout, ring cowbells and bang pots, play bagpipes and trombones as they line the streets of the New York City Marathon course through five distinctive boroughs: Staten Island, Brooklyn, Queens, Manhattan and the Bronx.

Spectators turn the Marathon into the largest annual tailgate party that not even college football, NFL or NASCAR can top. Parties begin in Brooklyn and carry on to Manhattan's Upper East Side, complete with champagne, bagels, lox and beer, featuring revelers who hang over balconies to glimpse the race. Churches send choirs or roll out the steel drums, setting up breakfasts and barbecues. Communities hold bake sales on the sidewalk. Students and alumni from high schools perform outdoor concerts.

Fans admire the athletes who blur by them and those who shuffle past. They hold fluorescent posters and hang sheet banners for friends and family along the route, making runners feel like stars. Kinship marks the day, especially for the recreational runner who gets to compete on the same course and cross the same finish line as the professional.

Marathons have become remarkably accessible in the last two

decades, and even more so with the proliferation of entries allotted to charities. From funding cancer research to supporting school programs that aim to reduce obesity, charity pledge programs have given runners motivation beyond themselves, and this has sparked the latest running boom.

It is widely accepted that the American marathoner Frank Shorter ignited the distance running craze by winning the gold medal in the marathon at the 1972 Munich Olympics. The second, more populous movement began because of a milestone birthday. In 1995, Oprah Winfrey ran the Marine Corps Marathon in celebration of her fortieth birthday (finishing in 4:29:20), and motivated other first-timers to compete despite not having the prototype runner's body.

Fred Lebow, who cofounded the New York City Marathon in 1970, believed anybody could access the power of running. A Holocaust survivor from Romania, Lebow was, until he died of brain cancer in 1994, an indefatigable champion of the race he created, insisting it could transform lives.

As president of the New York Road Runners club, the organization founded in 1958 that directs the race, Lebow and his bearded, animated face made New York's Marathon famous throughout the world. The first race was held in Central Park with 127 runners, with only one woman among them. Six years later, by 1975, the Marathon grew to 534 runners, and soon after, talk began of widening the race to all five boroughs in the city. George Spitz, a city auditor and an active member of the Road Runners, first proposed the idea of timing the race to coincide with the nation's bicentennial. Even Lebow initially had to be talked into endorsing the wild idea of shutting down the city for an amateur athletic competition.

On Sunday morning, October 24, 1976, 2,090 runners had paid their five-dollar entrance fee and showed up at Fort Wadsworth in

Staten Island to start the race on the Verrazano-Narrows Bridge. Like the runners, Lebow had approached the day with equal parts trepidation and anticipation.

"I think Fred hoped it would change the face of marathoning," said Tucker Andersen, 65, who ran that first race in 1976 and has run every year since. "But who knew?"

Not even Lebow could have predicted that the New York City Marathon would grow to such a phenomenon that thirty-two years later more than 100,000 people would apply for entry into the race lottery and less than half would be accepted. Or that the Marathon would come to generate revenues of more than $200 million a year for New York.

The race has gone on every year, in rain, heat or wind, the event itself serving as testament to perseverance. In November 2001, only seven weeks after the September 11, 2001, terrorist attacks, more than 25,000 runners started the race in front of a 150-foot-tall banner—"United We Run"—created in solidarity by the Berlin Marathon five weeks earlier. New Yorkers and runners from most nations on the globe wore red, white and blue, as they slapped hands with firemen and policemen along the route for an emotional tribute.

Since 2003, the Netherlands-based financial services company ING has been the race's title sponsor—a necessity in the twenty-first-century professional sports landscape—enabling the New York Road Runners to showcase their premier event worldwide and attract elite talent. With an enthusiastic and personal touch, Mary Wittenberg, the 45-year-old Road Runners' chief executive and president, has recruited aggressively and sought to help fund emerging talent in the United States. She wants to popularize the sport of distance running by marketing runners as if they were superstars of the NBA or Major League Baseball.

Wittenberg was the whirlwind force behind bringing the 2008

United States Men's Olympic Marathon Trials to New York and pairing the race with the New York City Marathon. At cocktail parties, lunches and press conferences leading up to the double header, Wittenberg talked herself hoarse while promoting the "greatest marathon weekend in history."

Privately, though, she was nervous. International marathons in 2007 had been beset by oddities and bad weather, from the nor'easter that blew through Boston in April 2007 to the heat-induced disaster in Chicago later that year. The 2007 Chicago Marathon, on October 7, had to be canceled after three hours, because the temperature reached a record high of 88 degrees for the race. Aid stations ran out of water. Medical tents were overflowing with runners, and 184 participants were taken to the emergency room. A 35-year-old Michigan police officer, Chad Schieber, died when he suffered a heart attack after the 18-mile mark.

Despite its thorough preparation, New York would not be immune to catastrophe. During the U.S. Olympic Trials on November 3, 2007, one day before New York's Marathon, Ryan Shay, a former national marathon champion, collapsed suddenly in Central Park after running only five and a half miles. Just 28, Shay was pronounced dead of cardiac arrest less than an hour later.

Shay's unassailable work ethic would become his legacy, but it would also prompt difficult questions. How hard can a runner push and why? Can this happen to anyone? Were performance-enhancing drugs involved? Some questions would remain unanswered even after the full autopsy results were released four months later showing that Shay died of natural causes.

Although marked by tragedy, the November 2007 Olympic trials also celebrated the emergence of young talent: Ryan Hall, 25, who gamely ran a trials record time of 2:09:02 in the hills of Central Park as he set his path for the 2008 Beijing summer games. The day would forever be remembered by the name *Ryan*. One day later, the thirty-eighth New York City Marathon completed the back-to-back drama—two races framed by the competing forces of marathon history.

Were it not for a death, after all, this race and all of its glory never would have existed.

Pheidippides, an Athenian herald, supposedly ran 150 miles in two days to request help from Sparta, then raced a final 25 miles from the Marathon battlefield to Athens to announce the under-manned Greek victory over the Persians in 490 B.C.

"We have won!" Pheidippides proclaimed. And promptly dropped dead.

The first modern Olympics in Athens, in 1896, re-created his victory run (the official marathon distance of 26.2 miles was insti-tuted at the 1908 London Olympics), and in Greece today Pheidip-pides is still considered a folk hero.

Each major international marathon has since developed its own legacy, its own distinct identity. Established in April 1897, the Boston Marathon owns the tradition as the longest-running marathon in the world, with strict qualifying times for entry and an intimate racing atmosphere. The Chicago Marathon, histori-cally a competitor of New York in the same autumn season, is a flat course that encourages fast times (weather permitting). The same goes for Berlin, where Ethiopia's Haile Gebrselassie set the men's world record (2:04:26) in September 2007. The London Marathon, modeled after New York and started in 1981, is home to the wom-en's record, which the UK's Paula Radcliffe set in 2003 (2:15:25). London is also known for its fast course, one that draws top-flight professional fields as well as amateurs in outlandish costumes run-ning for charity.

New York, with its hidden hills and obvious inclines on and off the five bridges, may no longer produce the world's fastest times, but it offers instead an experience beyond just a road race. This is a day that is large, loud and unforgettable. Ordinary people become celebrities, and celebrities can feel the pain of ordinary people. For those who endure the grueling training, they earn T-shirts, music, medals and parties, and over the course of 26.2 miles, a citywide standing ovation.

Only four professional athletes—one male and one female runner, and one male and one female wheelchair racer—can break the tape in Central Park and wear the handmade laurel crown. Everyone else shares the glory of completing a goal.

Fast and slow, old and young, untested and undaunted, those who participate, volunteer or cheer form a bond for one day. This simple act of running, putting one foot in front of the other fast, ultimately connects people and completes them.

To be sure, the Marathon is not an idyllic event, just as New York is not always the picture on the postcard. The race can be as raw as a heel blister, as unpredictable and as maddening as gridlocked Manhattan traffic. But for those other moments on the five-borough course when the crowds are roaring, the sun is dancing, the masses are rushing in rhythm and the endorphins kick in for an emotional turboblast known as a runner's high, the possibilities are exhilarating. In these unforgettable moments, the journey becomes the destination.

1

HUDDLED MASSES

The Start, Fort Wadsworth, Staten Island

One hundred and forty buses line Midtown Manhattan in the hazy darkness before dawn, idling for a mass evacuation to Staten Island.

As streams of sleepy runners shuffle through the unblinking glare of headlights, they follow instructions spit from the megaphones of men and women wearing orange jackets. This apocalyptic activity might seem unusual—even for New York—were it not the first Sunday in November.

The thirty-eighth running of the New York City Marathon will start in five hours, and Pam Rickard is anxious, holding her husband Tom's hand as she prepares to board her bus. Tom has faithfully accompanied his wife of 21 years from the foothills of the Blue Ridge Mountains to the steps of the New York Public Library on Fifth Avenue and 42nd Street. The caravan awaits her. When they approach the door to one of the buses, a man lowers his megaphone and looks at Tom.

"This is where you kiss her good-bye," he says sternly. "You're not going any farther."

A lump catches in Pam's throat. She heard those exact words in September 2006 when she walked into the Roanoke County jail to complete her 90-day sentence for driving under the influence of alcohol, the punishment for her third offense in two years.

Fourteen months later, she is going to run her eighth marathon. It is her first in New York and the first since she became sober. Pam is 45 years old, a 5-foot-6 mother of three daughters with wavy black hair and a perfectly toned runner's body. But the faint wrinkles around her eyes reveal the hard living she fought so long to hide and the new life she is fighting even harder to maintain. Her jaw is taut in determination.

Last year on this very Sunday, she was collecting trash by the side of Virginia Route 581, wearing an orange jumpsuit and hoping no one would recognize her. Today, she wears an orange bib with the number F5079 and revels in her anonymity.

When Pam learned she had won a number from the New York City Marathon lottery back in June, she was humbled by the odds she had beaten. Of the 43,989 U.S. residents who had applied, she was one of 8,157 accepted. She does not want to forsake her second chance.

In New York Harbor, the patron of second chances stands guard, welcoming the world to her shores. As the sun rises in ribbons of rose, gold and orange, marathoners peering out of buses or ferry windows easily spot the Statue of Liberty and her torch, forever lit. A mile away, on the northern tip of Staten Island, the masses of runners are beginning to huddle.

They emerge from an alphabet of origins, from Andorra to Venezuela and from Lake Michigan to Zoo Lake. New York may have been the destination for millions over the centuries, but the city represents only the beginning of a newcomer's journey. Simply arriving is not enough; achieving here is what matters. The soaring skyscrapers, majestic bridges and millions of people lining expansive (and expensive) avenues demand an effort of an equally epic scale.

Today will be no Sunday morning jog.

"Good morning! Welcome to Staten Island! Have a great race!" Mike Poirier shouts from his lawn chair on the concrete stoop of his small Bay Street house. Somnambulant figures step from the shuttle buses that had collected them at the Staten Island Ferry terminal and traipse past him.

When Poirier bought his house nine years ago, the real estate agent neglected to tell him that the biggest event in the city's calendar would pass by his front door every November. Unshaven and wearing his U.S. Army Retired baseball cap, Poirier happily sips the coffee his wife hands him and shouts out the same greetings to waves of runners.

Poirier's house is just outside the grounds of Fort Wadsworth, which sits at the base of the soaring Verrazano-Narrows Bridge. The fort is one of the longest operating military defense strongholds in the country, protecting New York Harbor for nearly 200 years. Officially completed in 1865, it originally housed troops from the Army and then from the Navy until 1994, when the Coast Guard moved into the barracks. Men went off to World War II after training at Fort Wadsworth, and Nike missiles were stocked in hidden batteries throughout its grounds during the Cuban Missile Crisis. Today, the fort will host people going off to a different kind of battle.

For the better part of five hours, the grounds will turn into a self-sustaining village of approximately 50,000 people—an intricately planned operational marvel populated not only by the runners, but also volunteers, New York Road Runners staff, members of the media, entertainers and law enforcement officials from national and local agencies responsible for the safety and security of the event.

A New York Police Department patrol car escorts the bus that carries Harrie Bakst and his older brother, Rich, from Manhattan to Staten Island. They are part of the caravan of 12 buses carrying Fred's Team members, all running for the charity founded by Fred Lebow, the late founder of the New York City Marathon. Lebow established this team with the Memorial Sloan-Kettering Cancer Center in 1991, when he was being treated at the hospital for brain cancer. When Harrie was younger, he never thought he would run a marathon, much less be treated for cancer at Memorial Sloan-Kettering.

Harrie is 22 on race day, but he has always seemed to be an older soul, possessing a seriousness offset by his optimism. Cancer recently inscribed a story on his neck, leaving a violet, 4-inch scar just below the right side of his jaw.

In February 2007, Harrie went from being a robust senior at New York University, to a patient with adenoid cystic carcinoma, cancer of the salivary glands. During a routine checkup for a school trip to South Africa, a doctor felt a small lump in Harrie's neck, which turned into a life-changing diagnosis. After surgery to remove the tumor, Harrie underwent a grueling six-week course of radiation. It was then that Rich convinced him to run the New York City Marathon with these words:

"You're already going through the ultimate test of endurance," Rich said. "Next to that, the Marathon is a piece of cake."

Easy for Rich to say. He had already run the race in 2006 and knew what to expect. At 26, Rich, who stands 5 foot 10 and weighs 165 pounds, has a broad upper body but thin runner's legs. Harrie, dark-haired like his brother, is a solid 6-foot, 200 pounds, with a body that recalls his high school football and baseball days.

At the fort, the brothers disembark from the bus and make themselves comfortable with other Fred's Team members in the middle of a parking lot, chatting nervously in the impromptu circle. They help each other write their names on the team's purple-and-orange shirts and snap pictures to record the morning. Like many first-time marathoners—there are 15,722 of them here today—Harrie has heard the alarming stories about "The Wall." He has been told that an utter physical and mental depletion plagues the body somewhere after the 20-mile mark and makes runners feel as though they have run up against a concrete barrier and can go no farther. Harrie has run 20 miles, but no more, during any one training session. The uncertainty of how his body will react is Harrie's most overwhelming concern right now.

"Can I really do this?" he asks himself, echoing the unspoken refrain of virtually every other runner in the village.

Rich knows the Marathon will hurt his brother. It will hurt everybody in the race today. "But Harrie," Rich says, "is stronger than he thinks he is."

By 7:30 a.m., Fort Wadsworth is starting to generate kinetic energy. The guitars, drums and urgent vocals of the band, Blues BBQ, blast from the main soundstage like a radio alarm clock. The speakers spread through the village intone multilingual announcements—on a continuous loop in English, Spanish, Italian, German and Japanese—lending a distinctly Epcot Center feel to the morning.

Staten Island is the most overlooked of New York City's five boroughs, and the most suburban. Yet runners will spend as many (if not more) hours waiting here for the race to begin as they will running through the other four boroughs. Temperatures are in the high 40s, and to pass the time on this brisk morning, participants sit under layers of clothing and blankets.

The fortunate who belong to a charity team or who have connections to the race's premier sponsors can duck into heated tents stocked with pastries, fruit and beverages. Outside the hospitality tents, some runners rough it by camping out in sleeping bags, four bodies across, doing their best Woodstock impression. Those who did not think to bring enough layers lie in the fetal position to generate heat.

Other runners warm themselves by walking around and meeting new friends, swapping stories of why they are here and where they are from, taking care not to expend too much energy. Some sit silently by themselves at the base of trees, filling out the *New York Times* crossword puzzle or reading the Sunday paper, calming their anxiety by going through a routine. Others call loved ones, whose sleepy voices will ease their nerves.

Some runners are overjoyed to be here, having gained automatic entry after not being chosen in the lottery three times in a row. Others were guaranteed entry by the fast qualifying times they ran in a marathon or half-marathon in the previous year. But neither luck nor experience helps calm the jitters right now. One glance at the Verrazano-Narrows Bridge looming from every angle above the start village and the runners are reminded of the daunting task ahead.

As soon as they get to Fort Wadsworth, runners are directed to one of three distinct areas in the village that correspond to the color of their bib numbers: blue, green or orange. When the time comes, runners will proceed to corrals that direct them to the starting line on the bridge. Runners with blue and orange bibs will start on the bridge's upper deck, while those with green proceed to the lower deck.

Each distinct area of the village has the same characteristics—a massive arc of corral-colored balloons, first aid stations, and kiosks for coffee, tea, bagels and hot water. Runners queue for their prerace sustenance, but no line takes longer than five minutes. Due to complaints from 2006 participants who waited in lengthy lines to use portable toilets, 309 more were added in 2007 to the start village, bringing the total to 1,515.

The long lines will be elsewhere this year—at the parking lot where runners drop off their official clear plastic bags containing belongings not needed during the race; they will be deposited at numbered UPS trucks that correspond to their bib numbers. In the orange drop-off area, there is a gridlock of nearly one hour, as runners waiting to drop bags get caught in the exiting flow of those who already have done so. Nerves begin to fray in anticipation.

The pungent aroma of Bengay wafts unmistakably from the medical tents where runners try to ease their already tense muscles. Inside, runners also avail themselves of petroleum jelly, applying it to the body parts that will endure the most skin-on-skin friction. Men place Band-Aids over their nipples. Most marathoners have long eschewed the concept of modesty. But not all.

A few feet from the curb of the main street heading into the start village, a small open tent holds some forty men and five women, swaying and praying. Jewish marathoners from around the world spill out of the tent. Many drape prayer shawls over their running outfits and wrap tefillin (black boxes holding biblical inscriptions) on the arm and the forehead. Their mumbling grows to a crescendo at the morning minyan (a prayer gathering that traditionally had to have at least ten men), forming an intimate community within a community.

Around the corner, a tent ten times the size, with plastic windows lining its walls, offers ecumenical Christian services conducted by clerics who are themselves running the race. Cindy Peterson, who grew up Catholic in Montreal, cannot discern whether there will be a Mass this morning. No matter; she is there anyway to keep warm. Cindy and her teammates from the New York–based Mercury Masters have been wandering the fort since before sunrise. They belong to a team of women 50 years and older, but they are not the early-bird special types—unless it means getting up for a run. At 67, Cindy is the oldest Mercury Master running the race. It will be her twelfth New York City Marathon, her thirty-fifth marathon since she turned 55.

At 4 a.m., long before the group met in Manhattan for a picture, Cindy applied her champagne-colored lipstick, black eyeliner, tan eye shadow and foundation. She has platinum hair beneath her sparkling red-and-purple baseball cap, and she stands 5-foot–5, with a few extra grandmotherly pounds in the middle. Cindy looks as if she's ready for the stage, to sing as she did when she was a teenager in Canada. That was before her American ex-husband made her choose between him and her voice.

Cindy, who lives in Bedminster, central New Jersey, now travels freely around the globe to run marathons and partake of a growing, specialized tourist industry. On this day, however, the world comes to her backyard.

Foreign runners number 20,072 today and hail from 107 countries. Given that there are only 19,193 from the United States, this percentage—51 percent foreign—makes the New York City Marathon distinct. The ratio has always been typical of New York's race, while frustrating to local and U.S. runners applying. Early in the Marathon's five-borough history, Lebow made it his mission to recruit foreign runners to the most cosmopolitan city in the world. He befriended presidents of running clubs in France and Italy and those two countries, along with Great Britain and the Netherlands, still bring the most runners as part of tour groups. Most operators are filled to capacity eight months before the race.

"If you do one marathon on earth, you do this one," Peggy Sailler, of Saint-Malo, France, said one day before the race at the annual International Friendship Run. Nearly 15,000 runners gathered on the lawn outside the United Nations for the equivalent of an adult pep rally at 8:30 a.m., followed by a run through Midtown Manhattan that ordinarily would have taken them four miles, to Tavern on the Green, the famed Central Park restaurant where the Marathon finishes. This year, because the U.S. Olympic Marathon trials were being run in Central Park on Saturday morning, the course was only 1.7 miles long, so it was more of an "acquaintance run."

For some, that run was like a photo op with new running pals, a literal dress rehearsal. Today, for the actual performance, the costumes are out in force. A man and wife from Scotland wear matching purple wigs. A man in lederhosen holds a plastic beer glass attached to a tray. A woman from Japan wears a silk kimono, while another from France wears a tutu. Flocks of Italian-speaking runners stroll around in disposable heat-retaining polypropylene coveralls sold at the bustling Marathon Expo in the days before the race; they look as though they have just come from the night shift at a nuclear plant.

Superheroes are also patrolling the grounds, complete with cape and face paint, as if to advertise what running does for their self-image. One local favorite, Larry the Lighthouse (aka Darrin Goldman from New Jersey), fits inside a 5-foot Styrofoam lighthouse while he shuffles for charity. Just when you chuckle and think this odd mélange of characters must be extras from the Tatooine bar scene in *Star Wars*, Chewbacca shows up, with a bib number pinned to his fur. Naturally.

Far from the Carnavale that is the people's race, the sport's top international runners prepare in library silence. Their heated tent is located on the other side of the fort, beneath the southeast side of the bridge. There, the elite athletes have ample time to stretch and, later, warm up their legs on a long service road alongside softball fields.

By 8:30 a.m., Paula Radcliffe is staking her territory, stretching her hamstrings by setting her right leg atop a table next to a plate of croissants in the front of the tent. Her blue-green eyes sparkle in concentration, emitting a signal of absolute confidence. The other women try not to notice.

Radcliffe, 33 years old and born in Cheshire, England, holds the women's world marathon record she set in London in April 2003—2 hours, 15 minutes and 25 seconds. (She had shattered her own record of 2:17:18, which she ran in Chicago the previous October.) No woman since then, including Radcliffe, has come within three minutes of that eye-popping 2:15:25 mark.

Due to pregnancy and injury, she has not run a marathon since August 2005. Her first race back at any distance came at the Great North Run, a half-marathon in Newcastle, England, five weeks ago. Radcliffe finished a disappointing second place. The two-year layoff from competition was incredibly frustrating for her, but it did reap an incalculable reward—her daughter, Isla. Blond-haired, blue-eyed Isla has become a star at nine and a half months, happier in the limelight than her mother, who is a formidable, yet gracious superstar.

After Radcliffe kissed Isla good-bye to board the elites' bus leaving Manhattan this morning, she handed her daughter to her husband, Gary Lough. Isla waved to her mum sitting at the window inside the bus and then quickly lost interest, instead exploring new people around her. She spotted Getaneh Tessema, the husband of her mother's prime competition, Gete Wami, from Ethiopia. Isla wanted to be held by this kind man who always seems to be smiling. So Lough passed his daughter to Tessema, who bounced her in his arms; he missed his own four-year-old daughter, Eva, back in Addis Ababa.

The men remain in Manhattan to endure an anxious day. This is the thirty-third major race in which Radcliffe and Wami are competing against each other, but only the first at the marathon distance.

Wami, 32 years old, won the Berlin Marathon just 35 days earlier, running in front the entire time with a male pacesetter; no other woman was in contention after the first mile. That victory moved Wami into the lead for the inaugural $500,000 World Marathon Majors prize. A competition, which tabulates results over two years from marathons run in Boston, London, Berlin, Chicago and New York, concludes today. For the lure of this jackpot, Wami will attempt something so physically taxing that it is virtually unheard of in the sport; no man or woman has won major city marathons within five weeks of each other.

Wami looks nonplussed sitting at one of the round tables in the tent, as if she were attending a community breakfast. But this is how she appears while racing, too. Since Radcliffe did not run the last two years, Wami's primary competition today for the series prize money is Jelena Prokopcuka (pronounced pro-kup-CHU-ka), the two-time defending New York champion from Latvia.

Prokopcuka trails Wami by 10 points and must win the marathon outright or finish at least three spots ahead of Wami (but in no less than third place) to collect the half-million dollars.

An hour before the race, Prokopcuka is already warming up while trying to calm down. She knows her best times are not as fast as these other two women's. She also knows she could have a problem; a hip injury she sustained during a training run 35 days ago has not completely healed.

The marathon distance is nothing if not merciless. Those 26.2 miles—especially the final six, where the real race begins—have the ability to expose even the slightest of injuries and create new ones.

Professional runners pound the uneven pavement for more than two hours, taking an average of 190 steps per minute. Elite athletes will strike the ground about 25,000 times during the course of the race. Depending on their weight, they put more than 700 tons of impact stress on each leg during a single marathon.

Confidence, along with proper training, good health, good strategy, and, ultimately, luck, can soften the minute-by-minute blow and contribute to a successful marathon day. A runner needs a harmonic convergence of these factors and then perhaps also needs an opponent out of sync. Even then, breaking the tape first is not assured.

The distance, itself, is the most menacing foe of all.

"I am still afraid of the marathon," South Africa's Hendrick Ramaala admitted a few months before the race. "I think all the guys deep down, they know. They are scared of the marathon."

Ramaala speaks like a man who has lost more marathons than he has won—a professional not afraid to acknowledge he is mortal. In fact, he has won only two of the 20 marathons he has entered since 1999. He is his country's top marathoner, the 2004 New York champion and the infamous New York runner-up in 2005, when he lunged across the finish line and stumbled just three-hundredths of a second late.

At 35, aging by marathon standards, Ramaala is not yet ready to rest on his laurels.

Inside the tent that the elite men and women share, he speaks easily with the 29-year-old favorite from Kenya, Martin Lel, and nods to Morocco's Abderrahim Goumri, who at 31 is a relative upstart in the sport. In his debut marathon seven months ago in

London, Goumri engaged Lel to the final 300 meters—until he surged too soon and watched the veteran Lel confidently sprint past him to the finish line. Lel was born into the sport, belonging to Kenya's Kalenjin tribe, which has the majority of its country's star runners. Goumri's father, a mason from Morocco, did not accept that his son could make a living with his feet—until Goumri started winning national races.

Ramaala, a lawyer, is the only runner with an advanced degree in this collection of elite athletes, even though he has never practiced. He is well liked by his fellow athletes for his quick wit and his down-to-earth charm.

Professional runners, even with their 140-mile training weeks, their tolerance for pain and their extremely regimented schedules, are not so different from the recreational athletes. Today, they are all competitors, out to test themselves.

Hendrick Ramaala and Jelena Prokopcuka, Paula Radcliffe and Gete Wami, Martin Lel and Abderrahim Goumri, Pam Rickard, Harrie Bakst and Cindy Peterson are the archetypes of this race: a cancer survivor, a recovering alcoholic, a grandmother, intimidating champions and contenders trying to keep pace. Their stories tell of survival and reinvention, persistence and determination. The lives of these runners and their experiences on the course reflect the grandiose dreams and gritty challenges of New York, as well as the eclectic spirit of the city's distinct neighborhoods.

Not everyone starts the New York City Marathon with a poignant or compelling tale, but they can create one in the time it takes to run 26.2 miles.

The competitors chosen here serve as windows into a one-day festival of soles, guides to a journey of self-discovery that will unfold mile by mile.

2

EPIC ASPIRATIONS

Verrazano-Narrows Bridge

Five helicopters and a blimp hover like buzzards above the Verrazano-Narrows Bridge, pounding out a steady pulse. The heartbeats from the herd of 39,265 athletes echo below. Runners are assembling, elbow to elbow, in groups of 1,000, and they stream endlessly, it seems, onto the bridge's two decks to compete in the world's largest marathon.

By 9:30 a.m., runners are in line, stretching, laughing, befriending strangers, dancing to music from headphones, trying to stay warm, trying to stay positive, nervously bouncing on the balls of their feet, some even squatting and flushing their bodily fluids right there on the bridge as the minutes tick down to a day of certain torture.

The assault on the senses is typical New York. Here, the sheer volume of humans, smells, noises, accents, anxieties and ambitions is enough to overwhelm anyone, even those who think they are prepared. And even those who are no longer running.

It has been two decades since Norway's Grete Waitz captured her ninth and final New York City Marathon title, a record that no other runner can or likely will match. Sitting in the backseat of the red convertible pace car, where she will serve as the grand marshal of the women's professional race today, Waitz cannot help but feel the spark of Marathon electricity on the bridge this morning.

"Even now when I'm out there at the Verrazano, with the helicopters circling, I feel the goose bumps as if I'm going to compete," she says. "It's still the same feeling."

Alberto Salazar knows the feeling intimately—he won the New York City Marathon three consecutive years in the early eighties, and like Waitz, set a world record on the course. Salazar may first envision the finish line in New York, but when he considers the defining image of this Marathon, he turns back to the Verrazano-Narrows Bridge for its scene of breathtaking enormity.

"It's like a Cecil B. De Mille movie, because it's on such a huge, epic scale," Salazar said, reflecting some months before the Marathon. "It's like huge armies clashing. There are thousands of people, sirens, helicopters, pandemonium. There is no other event like it."

No matter that only a handful of competitors hope to win today. "It's not so much about beating other people," Salazar said, speaking for the masses. "You want to see how hard you can push yourself, who can take the most pounding."

Salazar, long removed from his running career at 48, recently provided a chilling reminder of the body's physical limits and, in his lucky case, its surprising capabilities. In July 2007, Salazar suffered a heart attack while training runners on the Nike campus in Beaverton, Oregon. His heart stopped for 14 minutes. He received immediate CPR, and paramedics shocked him eight times with defibrillators, eventually reviving him. Salazar, who has a family history of heart disease, had a blockage in his coronary artery. Doctors performed surgery and inserted a stent to open the artery and regulate his heartbeat. Three weeks before this year's New York City Marathon, doctors would find another blockage. Salazar, despite coaching runners who were entered in the Olympic trials, was not allowed to travel to New York this weekend.

Last year, Salazar accompanied Lance Armstrong, the seven-time Tour de France champion, during the opening 10 miles of Armstrong's much-ballyhooed first marathon.

"He went out too fast," Salazar recalled.

The 1984 Olympic marathon champion Joan Benoit Samuelson was also in Armstrong's entourage, elbowing curious runners out of the way in the final 10 miles as Armstrong winced his way to a 2:59:36 finish. Armstrong made climbing the Alps on a bicycle look routine. But he proclaimed the 2006 Marathon in New York his toughest physical experience, to the glee of some professionals and die-hard amateurs who did not want their sport to be taken lightly.

"I don't want to have another month like I did last year," Armstrong says today, standing on one leg. He is stretching his quadriceps after stepping out of his black SUV near the elite athletes' tent. "For a week, I couldn't walk."

He later learned that what he thought were shin splints were, in fact, stress fractures. He vowed to be better prepared this year. Armstrong is relieved not to have a "LanceCam" shadowing him for Internet consumption this time. Nor will he have an A-list of escorts.

Armstrong, at 5 foot 10, 173 pounds, is about 10 pounds lighter this year and in better shape, bitten by the bug that afflicts so many first-time marathoners. But with such painful memories of New York in 2006, why did he return?

"I like to have something in my life to keep me going," he says.

"The pressure of doing a marathon keeps me going, keeps me fit, and I can tie in the foundation work."

His survival from advanced testicular cancer at age 25 in 1996 was the impetus to form his cancer research charity, the Livestrong Foundation, and on this day, 130 members will be running as part of his team.

Armstrong returned to satisfy his restless competitive spirit, but he was also drawn back, he says, by the memory of New York's exuberant spectators, the intimate sidewalk give-and-take. "The fans, they don't just come out and cheer the leader, they just hang out. They're there all day, cheering everybody," Armstrong says, shaking his head in amazement. "Somebody who's not from here, you never know these boroughs, these neighborhoods exist. You go from one corner, and there's this Motley Crue cover band and on another corner, a bunch of Hasidic Jews. It's crazy."

New York's allure is the reason why rap star Sean "P. Diddy" Combs ran in 2003. It is also one reason why Katie Holmes, the 28-year-old actor and wife of Tom Cruise, contacted the Road Runners a few months before the race, requesting to run her first marathon.

At 5 a.m., a representative for Holmes woke up a New York Road Runners staff member and reported Holmes had lost her required bib and the timing chip that is attached to a runner's shoelaces. She would need one more of each. And, as pre-arranged, she was to be registered as Kate Smith.

Holmes was supposed to be on the elite athletes' bus, but when she did not show up in time, the bus left without her. Race organizers were told Holmes would get to the starting line on her own—an effort, presumably, to dodge the paparazzi. She does. She has two trainers doubling as bodyguards who plan to run with her, plus a crew of security following her throughout her run, waiting for her at each of the initial 18 first-aid stations along the course.

In the lead-up to the 2007 race, event organizers were too busy preparing for the Olympic trials to court other high-profile celebrities but welcomed them when they wanted to participate. Alex Zanardi, the Italian race car driver who lost both of his legs in a racing accident, is competing in the hand-cycle wheelchair division. Mike Richter, the retired New York Rangers goalie, is running in support of the charity operated by ING, "Run for Something Better," which promotes running in New York City schools. This is Richter's first marathon ever since finishing an Ironman triathlon in 2006.

"Suddenly you're 40 years old, and you're eating the same," Richter reflected days before the race. "I said to myself, 'Maybe I should get a program.'"

The running program led him to discover that the two sports were not so different. As a hockey goalie, he was always alone in front of the net, trying to stay focused while fighting through exhaustion.

"The essence of real athletes is that you're always competing against yourself," Richter said. "With running, it's just a different arena. That feeling I had when playing hockey, it's still there. You play with as much excellence as you can."

Race director Mary Wittenberg understands that concept of perfectionism. Since before sunrise she has been racing all over Fort Wadsworth and the Verrazano-Narrows Bridge, conducting television interviews, overseeing the operations of the start village and meeting sponsors with a smile—an event planner in her element. She climbed over the barricades to greet the wheelchair athletes assembling adjacent to the bridge and then sprinted down the hill to the elite athletes' tent, where she greeted the professionals and also met with Armstrong and New York City Mayor Michael

Bloomberg, who arrived via helicopter. Then she retreated to the command center trailer on the bridge, where she printed important phone numbers and course records on a pink Post-it pad that she would affix to the back of the credentials hanging from her neck.

With an indefatigable will, a runner's rail-thin body and a passion for the athletes in her races, Wittenberg, 45, created a career in a sport that once rejected her. She had wanted to be a runner when she was growing up as the oldest of seven children in Buffalo, New York. She was cut from the track team three times, but Wittenberg discovered at Canisius College in Buffalo that she had the endurance and the mental resolve to excel as a competitive rower and a coxswain.

Wittenberg got her chance to compete as a runner when, with only a year of eligibility left, she joined the cross-country team at Notre Dame as a first-year law student. She started training for marathons despite demanding work hours as a first-year law associate in Richmond, Virginia. In 1988, she won the Marine Corps Marathon. Her time—2 hours, 44 minutes and 36 seconds—was a good 20 minutes off an elite-level pace, but it qualified her for the 1988 women's Olympic Trials. A back injury cut short Wittenberg's Olympic bid just two miles into the trials.

"Part of me always wonders how good I could have been," Wittenberg said. "I'm very comfortable because I don't think I would have been that good.

"Most of us who run, we have personalities that we're either going to be the best or we're going to do something else."

This is a day that ends with a celebration of individual achievement; the start recognizes those individuals with the courage to be here in the first place. Giovanni da Verrazano was the first

European to sail through these narrow waters in 1527. Othmar H. Ammann, the Swiss-born engineer, outdid himself by creating a bridge to span what Verrazano had discovered. It was Ammann's sixth and final bridge in New York City, and it was considered his masterpiece; construction was made possible by Robert Moses, New York's "master builder" and premier city planner. Moses overcame decades of political resistance and neighborhood protests to see the bridge finally connect Staten Island and Brooklyn on November 21, 1964.

Weighing nearly 1.3 million tons, the bridge has two decks and a maximum of twelve traffic lanes that approximately 200,000 vehicles use daily. It spans 4,620 feet (a little less than a mile), making it the longest suspension bridge in North or South America—surpassing San Francisco's Golden Gate Bridge. Today, the 39,000 runners will feel a slight movement while crossing the span, as if they are bouncing softly on the springs of a mattress.

Jim Fortunato, who spent twelve years as the bridge's general manager, has a unique perspective on the structure, which has been something of a big brother to him, ushering him through life. On the bridge's Brooklyn-side promenade, also known as Lovers Lane, Fortunato once walked with his high school girlfriend, Joan. "Remember all the times we spent over here," Jim wrote to Joan, his words stretching across a picture of the bridge that was on the inside of his 1972 Fort Hamilton High School yearbook.

When Fortunato and Joan were married in 1975, they made the bridge the background for their wedding pictures. By then, Jim had left the bridge's Staten Island–side toll booth—his first job at age 16. Now, at 53, Fortunato serves as the Chief Command Center officer for a race defined by his life's love.

"The Bridge *is* the Marathon," Fortunato said. "It's the shot seen 'round the world."

This is the shot broadcast internationally on November 4, 2007: The morning sun glistens off the glassy harbor, illuminating a scene dotted with ships up to the Hudson River and out to the Atlantic Ocean. When the New York Fire Department boats spray water in three fountains of red, white and blue at the start of the race, it is a sight so awesome that not even a camera lens can capture its scale. Only the runner on the bridge can truly appreciate its grandeur.

Joanne Navarra does have an impressive view, however, 90 feet in the air. She is in the tower of the fire rescue truck in front of the toll booths, overseeing the flow of foot traffic and the start operations. This was the invention her husband, Vic, a former New York firefighter, called his eye in the sky.

Victor Navarra can no longer see, because sinus tumors have blinded him. Confined to a wheelchair, he is not waiting to die. He lives for the Marathon start he has organized since 1982.

In 1980, Navarra, a Staten Island athletic club president, was unable to train for the Marathon after breaking his ribs fighting a fire, so he became a race volunteer at Lebow's insistence. Two years later, Navarra had become the coordinator for the start, involving friends, Staten Island neighbors and his family. He soon became an innovative force in the marathon industry, popularizing the corral system that feeds thousands of runners into different chutes onto the bridge.

His daughter April is caring for him today while his other daughter, Kristie, directs the operations with Joanne. His granddaughter, Marissa Madson, nine, is working the starting line.

Two months earlier, Navarra rattled off race-related details that made him most proud, including the 28,000 cups of coffee served each year in the start village. "The Marathon is my passion, my love and my excitement," Navarra said.

Navarra retired as a firefighter in 1999, robustly healthy at age

47. But on September 12, 2001, a day after his Engine Company 40 and Ladder 35 from Manhattan's Upper West Side lost thirteen men in the World Trade Center terrorist attacks, he was back on duty. He worked at ground zero for three straight months and it was there, he and Joanne believed, that he was exposed to toxic fumes that caused his cancer.

Doctors told Navarra in April 2007 that he likely had three months to live. So when October came, Vic and Joanne discussed their toughest contingency question for the start: What if he were to die right before the 2007 Marathon?

"He told me, 'The Marathon will go on, and we will have the funeral when we are finished,'" Joanne recalled three weeks before the race.

As organizers were girding themselves for his death, though, it was the unexpected tragedy that rocked the weekend.

Navarra felt an icy shiver when Joanne told him about Ryan Shay's heart attack in Saturday's Olympic trials. The couple remembered how Shay had won the 5-mile Pepper Martin Run in Staten Island on July 4, 2001—a time when both men had been spirited and carefree.

Vic Navarra would die on December 30, 2007, at age 55. A man eager to guide others onto the right path, Navarra would want people to dwell not on the ending, but, as always, on the beginning.

Today's race marks a new beginning in Pam Rickard's life. She wears an old sweatshirt that belonged to her brother-in-law, Jimmy, who died of cancer in February 2006. Standing in the corral with runners speaking foreign languages makes Pam feel as though she is at the Olympics. But the next moment, she suddenly feels alone, flooded with fear, grief and guilt. She feels she does not deserve to be part of such a celebratory event after the pain she caused her family.

"I should have waited and done it next year," she thinks.

Pam takes a deep breath and remembers the mantra of the 12-step recovery program of Alcoholics Anonymous. It is a power larger than she is. *I have done all I can to prepare*, she thinks. *I have to surrender to the Marathon.*

Besides, Pam cannot back out now. There is no way she could squeeze through the massive crowds and get off the bridge. And her husband, Tom, is waiting for her in Manhattan.

Pam takes off the sweatshirt on the way to the bridge and hangs it on a fence alongside other clothing, in memory of Jimmy and her former self. A Girl Scout troop from New Jersey will help gather clothing from Fort Wadsworth while others will scavenge for the best items left behind, from running tights to iPods. The items discarded on the bridge, however, will likely not be given to charity. In order for clothes to be donated, they must be washed. The volume of clothing, mixed with trash and even runners' urine, is just too great for the Department of Sanitation trucks to separate before the bridge must reopen in two hours.

Today, the last runner will not reach the starting line until after 11 a.m. The majority of the runners take an average of 30 minutes to get there, but at least the timing chip on their sneakers records the net time, from the instant they cross the starting line to the instant they cross the finish line. The wait to get to the start will be interminable for some who have been in Staten Island for nearly five hours.

After months of grueling training, enduring rainstorms and blackened toenails, long runs and hill work, runners are anxious to begin their quest. What will they learn about themselves? How far will they push?

Harrie turns to his brother, Rich, and says, "26.2." They pound their fists in the family handshake and get ready to cross the bridge.

At 10:05 a.m., the sun is now golden and strong, the air just as invigorating at 53 degrees and the winds whispering at 5 miles an hour—ideal conditions for running a marathon. The elite runners are assembled at the line, and when each is introduced, the masses behind them and to their left cheer heartily.

A few feet behind the male professional runners (the women professionals have started 35 minutes earlier) stand the elite runners from New York City's fire and police departments—the police dressed in royal blue singlets, the firemen in engine red. For the past 25 years, the two departments have had a serious (and sponsored) team competition for the Mayor's Cup, fielding more than 200 combined runners. They have work to do before they can run, however. Since 1992, when the Marathon had a false start, more than a dozen top police and fire department runners have lined up at the front of the people's race, linking arms to prevent anyone from jumping out in front until the cannons signal the start.

The runners and the spectators on the grandstand join city and race officials and officers in uniform on the bridge to create an atmosphere of tingling anticipation. And then, abruptly, the buzz stops when the national anthem singer (Tevin Campbell from the musical *Hairspray*) steps to the stage.

His first few familiar notes transform the morning into a sporting event, officially bringing amateur runners into the big time. Those from the United States place their hands over their hearts and many sign along. Men and women take off their caps. The runners turn toward the flag, facing lower Manhattan, nearly in line with where the World Trade Center towers once stood. For those who are not so far back in the crowd to hear, the moment brings chills to even the most warmly dressed runners. After the final notes of the "Star-Spangled Banner," some 39,000 amateur runners scream at the top of their lungs, releasing their excitement . . . or their anxiety.

It is 10:10 a.m. and Mary Wittenberg, her throat crackling from a sleepless night grieving for Shay, now takes the microphone. After asking for a moment of silence in Shay's memory, Wittenberg implores the runners to make this a day of healing. "We wish each of you the race of a lifetime," she shouts.

"The city is all yours today! Are you ready to run?"

The pair of 75-millimeter howitzer cannons sitting on a U.S. Army truck in the middle of the bridge boom like thunder as two puffs of ashy smoke float into a cloudless sky.

Frank Sinatra starts spreading the news, the sound system blasting his rendition of "New York, New York." No matter how corny it may sound, the song has become a hallmark of the New York City Marathon send-off, an anthem unto itself.

Marathoners come from around the world "to be a part of it" and to finish at "the top of the heap," to borrow from the song's famous words. Surely as motivational tunes go, Sinatra's reminder of making it in New York fuels an empowering possibility.

Today is, indeed, a brand-new start.

3

FAIRY-TALE BEGINNING

Women's Professional Start

Paula Radcliffe is poised on the line, her ears attuned to the starter's horn as if she were in the blocks for a 100-meter race. For a relentless perfectionist like Radcliffe, every meter counts, even when there are 42,195 of them.

She is feeling that familiar rush of confidence and adrenaline again on the starting line, a refreshing tonic following her two-year absence from the sport. Her heart, which will pound out a steady 180 beats per minute in the next two-plus hours on the course, is revving like an engine from its resting rate of 38 beats per minute.

At 9:35 a.m., the horn signals the beginning of the professional women's marathon, and Radcliffe takes the first auspicious step— already a split-second ahead of the field.

Falling in behind Radcliffe, the 37 other professional women form a silent but powerful minority as they march uphill to the crest of the bridge. The women's start was not always this way. In 1972, the six women participating in the New York City Marathon sat in protest because they were required to start 10 minutes before the men. After that, the sexes started simultaneously. But in 2002, marathon organizers realized it would be a boon to have women start 35 minutes before the elite men and the masses, thereby maximizing television exposure.

True, the elite women miss out on the company and some of the ceremony—no cannon signals their start, no fireboats spray in the harbor and Frank Sinatra does not sing until later. Charlotte Cohn (of the Broadway musical *La Boheme*) belts out "God Bless America" before the horn goes off. But for athletes accustomed to grinding out two-hour training runs in mountainous terrain, such pomp is of little consequence, especially if they get to run the streets by themselves.

Radcliffe and her competitors surge to the peak of the Verrazano-Narrows Bridge, the highest elevation on the course today, at 260 feet above sea level and a dizzying 225 feet above shimmering New York Harbor. By the time they are one mile into the race—a little more than halfway over the bridge—the runners accelerate to a 5-minute, 42-second pace. The women are too busy monitoring a checklist of their bodies' initial responses to register the song blasting from the speakers on the bridge. Rod Stewart's "Hot Legs" is so inappropriate for the occasion that it just might be appropriate.

Possessing a rock-solid body and a blistering turnover, the modern female professional marathoner—mother, wife and champion—takes the center of the Brooklyn-bound roadway. The toll has already been paid.

Paula Radcliffe, Gete Wami, Jelena Prokopcuka and Catherine Ndereba are the most decorated in the field today. Each has an enlightened husband who supports and trains with her. Only Prokopcuka, who is 31 and the youngest of this group, is not yet a mother. The other three women each have daughters; Jane Ndereba is the eldest at ten. Her mother's nickname is Catherine the Great, and as the reigning world champion from Kenya at age 35, Ndereba has established a benchmark for women in Africa to be successful as mothers as well as professional athletes.

These four champions have built houses with their winnings, provided for their families, secured lucrative shoe company contracts, set records and become stars in their countries.

Today, each has a strategy to add to that cache. But each woman has a vulnerability, too.

Ndereba wants to see how she endures the early pounding to her legs, and whether her body has fully recovered from winning the world championship marathon in the oppressive heat of Osaka, Japan, eleven weeks earlier. She is the only woman in the world besides Radcliffe to have run faster than 2 hours, 19 minutes, but that was back in 2001, when Ndereba won the Chicago Marathon in 2:18:47.

Wami, who only five weeks ago won the Berlin Marathon, knows she may not surprise Radcliffe at the end of the race as she did in their earlier memorable duels. But Wami, who has never taken an early lead in races (preferring to surge at the end, which is the Ethiopian style) intends to stay on Radcliffe's heels.

Radcliffe retreats behind her dark sunglasses, connecting to the road beneath her like an old friend. She checks her legs and confirms they are acting what she calls "normal." No pain. Only lightness. Flooded with giddy relief, Radcliffe now looks forward to the rest of the race. She charges to the front and plans to stay there, never looking back. That is how her father, Peter, taught her to compete when she was a child.

Prokopcuka is close to Radcliffe, off to her left on the bridge. Her bib number 1 and her uniform color—the orange and blue corporate colors of title sponsor ING—mark her position as the two-time defending champion. On each hip, Prokopcuka bears two No.1 stickers, one of which masks the precise area of concern.

Within the first 100 meters of the incline, stabbing pain goes off like an alarm in Prokopcuka's left hip. *Manage the pain*, Prokopcuka tells herself. *Stay as close as possible to Paula, at least until she runs away with a pace that is simply not possible for me.*

The fairy tale is not over yet.

O nce upon a time there was a young girl from the outskirts of Riga, the capital of Latvia. She loved her life. She had forests to run in, the Baltic Sea to swim in, wonderful friends to play with and a mother who thought her daughter hung the moon. Soon she had a husband who coached her and completed her sentences the same way he completed her soul.

Jelena Prokopcuka never knew she was looking for something until she found it.

She and her husband, Aleksander Prokopcuks, who had retired as Latvia's top male marathoner, went to Switzerland in 2005 to train at altitude for the New York City Marathon. One day, they decided to build their workout around a run to a mountain lake that they located on a map. They ran for an hour. No lake. They ran another hour. No lake. During the third hour, they were not happy. Stubbornly, the couple kept searching.

Finally, their eyes caught a light coming from a clearing. It was a lake the size of a pond. They turned to each other with the same dumbfounded look and laughed. *This is what we came for?* They took some black rocks from the lake—not to remember the destination, but what Prokopcuka discovered on the journey: the value of pain and perseverance.

"After that," Aleks said, "Jelena wins New York."

He and his wife told the story while looking at the trophy case in their apartment in Jurmala, the Russian-populated resort town on the Baltic Sea that is 20 minutes from Riga. Four glass shelves glistened with sterling silver chalices from his and her competitions, medals, marathon bibs from New York and a dried laurel crown. There, on the middle shelf were the rocks from St. Moritz.

The stories Prokopcuka spins in her rapidly improving English are full of metaphor and have the lyrical quality of the fairy tales she adored while growing up in her Russian-speaking home, where Alexander Pushkin's stories for children were required reading.

She loved the story her mother told of the monster that captured a beautiful woman and the dashing young man who had to rescue her. He breaks in seven pairs of shoes while traveling over seven seas and through seven forests. In order to kill the monster, the young man must find a weapon that is hidden in the tree trunk, inside which is a rabbit, inside which is a duck, inside which is a needle. He snaps the needle in half, and the monster is magically killed.

Prokopcuka and her older brother, Andrei, did not grow up inside such a fantasyland, but rather in communist Latvia. For their parents, Vladimir and Valentina Celnova, the controlling Soviet state did provide some comforts. They could send their daughter to running camps, funded entirely by the government. They could live in their state-supplied apartment and share vodka with friends. When Communism fell and Latvia elected a democratic government in the shaky months of 1991, Prokopcuka was 15. Her parents, scrambling to cover finances, had to pay for camps and competitions. But otherwise, they made sure Jelena's life barely changed.

Sixteen years later, Prokopcuka has the life her mother wanted for her daughter, if not for herself.

"It was always my dream to have a house by the sea," Valentina said in Russian, as she stroked her daughter's soft dark brown hair in their apartment in suburban Riga. Six weeks before the New York City Marathon, Valentina was serving guests her homemade apple cider, fruit and cakes. Aleks's mother, Nadeja, made a blissfully rich batch of éclairs which she packed in one of her daughter-in-law's Nike shoe boxes.

In September 2007, the couple was putting the finishing touches on their dream house in Jurmala. Back in 2004, they bought three contiguous plots of land and then broke ground in July 2006. Prokopcuka won her first marathon in Osaka in March 2005, and by September 2007 her two New York titles were supporting the house's foundation.

"This house is a . . . monument of my success," she said, after searching for the right English words.

Prokopcuka walked inside the unfinished entry hall, and her husband wrenched off her stylish olive green leather boots from her pencil-thin jeans, an ensemble she bought in New York. Standing 5 foot 6 and weighing a lithe 114 pounds, she proudly offered a tour of her elegant Scandinavian-style house one late September day. Light woods and sleek dark furniture adorned the downstairs living room. The upstairs bedroom walls were painted with a texturing technique that took months. The state-of-the-art kitchen overlooked the lawn that would soon feature trees and a fountain. Eventually, there would be a long, paved driveway to the street. "To pay for this road, I have to win another New York," Prokopcuka joked.

There was also the little matter of tearing down the eyesore abutting the property—a two-level shanty in which an old man supposedly had died the previous year. "Soviet construction," she said, shaking her head.

The house, situated on a cozy block a half-mile from ritzy Kapu (Dune) Street, which is next to the Baltic Sea, was less expensive than the extravagant new mansions near the beach. For nine years, she and Aleks had lived a mile away in a cramped one-bedroom,

650-square-foot apartment that the Soviet government had given Aleks's father, Sergei, decades earlier.

Aleks's parents had moved across the street to an identical apartment complex. Aleks's mother, Nadeja, was a national champion cyclist for Belarus before moving to Latvia, and she passed on her competitive spirit and natural ability to Aleks. He still holds the national marathon record (2:15:56 in 1995) and was the country's top triathlete before coaching his wife.

Prokopcuka's mother-in-law and mother share a not-so-secret wish about the new house, which has three bedrooms. "I like the pink room," her mother, Valentina, said with a broad smile and a wink. "That's a nice room."

Her daughter rolled her eyes ever so slightly and nodded. There would be plenty of time to make that a baby's room.

"I think about it seriously," Prokopcuka would say later, out of her mother's home. "My mother and Aleks's mother, they talk about it for many, many years. In our country, they usually had a baby at age of 22 or 23, so this is too late for them. We are a new generation.

"It's very personal, because I have to decide when and why. It's not for my mother's and Aleks's mother. It wasn't like, 'you must.' It's my decision. They understand I have my career."

That career began innocently. As a child, Prokopcuka was in constant motion, so her mother took her to gymnastics and dancing classes. She was afraid to fall off the gymnastics apparatus and preferred "orienteering" in the forests of Riga with her classmates—"running with a compass," she termed it. At age 11, she was chosen to join the school track team, which seemed fun, for a while.

"I like it, but it was very difficult to go to training every day," Prokopcuka said. "I want to be with my friends in the yard."

One day she did not go to practice, and later the coach made a visit to the house. He informed her parents that while others could skip practice, their daughter must come every day, because she needed to develop her burgeoning talent. "We agreed with the coach that she needed to go to training, but we knew we could not make her with force," Vladimir recalled.

"It was my decision," Prokopcuka said. What changed her mind? "I won a local race and decided, 'I like winning.'"

At national competitions, Aleks remembered seeing this girl named Jelena, who was not so serious about running nor in shape. Two years later, he thought differently. "I see a very slim, beautiful woman, no teenager," he recalled. "When she was 20, it started getting serious."

The couple married three years later, in 1999, and Aleks took over from her first coach, Leonid Strekalovsky. Her results improved dramatically. In 2004, she became the Latvian champion in the 10,000 meters and in 2006 she won the national 3,000 meter title.

When did her mother know her daughter had talent?

"All the time!" Valentina declared.

To his wife's annoyance, Vladimir answered more literally. He first saw his daughter's talent emerge in 1996, he said, when she qualified for the Atlanta Olympics at age 19. She did not make the final of the 5,000 meters. Four years later, she finished ninth in the 5,000-meter final at the 2000 Sydney Games.

When asked about Prokopcuka's bid to become the first woman since the legendary Norwegian runner Grete Waitz to win three straight New York City Marathons, Prokopcuka's parents stared blankly, unfamiliar with this Waitz woman. "For them," Aleks explained in English, "the history of New York City Marathon starts when Jelena starts."

A poster of her crossing the finish line to win New York in 2006 is taped to the wall in her parents' spare room. Aleks's mother has a similar poster in her apartment from 2005, taped high and a little crookedly on an otherwise blank wood-paneled wall. Their families would be watching the 2007 race live on Eurosport at the house of Prokopcuka's brother, Andrei.

She tried her best not to raise expectations back home; the last year had been unsettling. She had bronchitis in February, which hampered her training for the Boston Marathon (she finished second). In July, Aleks's father died suddenly of a heart attack, and they rescheduled their summer training in St. Moritz for early September.

Sergei had been retired for 12 years and used to buy every newspaper and magazine that chronicled the careers of Aleks and Jelena. "He was my cheerleader," Prokopcuka said a week after the funeral. "He was a very kind man. Right now, running is my friend."

Just as she was getting back into a rhythm with her training in late September, she developed the hip injury on September 30. That was the same day that Wami was winning her marathon in Berlin and Radcliffe, in her first race back from pregnancy, was finishing second at the Great North Run half-marathon in England.

Prokopcuka had run 35 kilometers of a 38-kilometer run when she suddenly felt excruciating pain in her left hip muscle. She stopped and was unable to train the next day. After consulting a doctor, she chose the path of most resistance.

"I had to have my workouts, serious and hard," she explained. "Sometimes I felt this pain. Not to do? Or not to feel pain? Sometimes I had to take the decision on how I am feeling. I am still doing my workouts, because it's better. Each runner has the same problem."

An ultrasound showed damage to the muscle in the hip joint, but it was an injury that Aleks termed "a small injury, an inflammation."

She pushed through her workouts when she returned to Latvia, availing herself of extra massage therapy. In the late afternoon hours between her two-a-day, two-hour training sessions, she and Aleks would drive to the new house and talk with landscapers and architects and inspect the security system. The house was a welcome distraction.

"I'm only 31 and I have a house," Prokopcuka said. "We are very satisfied. We do not want for anything."

There is serenity in her, reflected in the glassy blue Baltic Sea, and there is security in her, reflected in the tall pines just off the beach. Between these two distinct natural features of Latvia, Jelena Prokopcuka lives comfortably, rooted in her identity.

Like any professional runner in tune with her body, she knows her limits. She has never beaten Radcliffe at any distance in their careers. Her personal best in the marathon is 2:22:56, more than seven minutes slower than Radcliffe's world record. Prokopcuka only hoped Radcliffe might not be as dominant in her first marathon in 15 months.

"Paula is Paula. I think she will push the pace," she predicted days before the race, adding one caveat. "Paula is not the real Paula—now she's almost equal. It's not like three years ago, when she ran 2:15, it was so unequal. She was so strong, so unbelievable."

Would the past be prologue for today's race? As soon as Prokopcuka peels off her snow-white arm warmers just past the first-mile mark on the bridge and heads toward the ramp to Brooklyn, she is already staring at Paula Radcliffe's back.

4

A DELIBERATE PATH

Men's and Mass Start, the Bridge to Bay Ridge

Hendrick Ramaala flashes a smile and does a double thumbs-up when the television camera stops in front of him. He is the only professional runner to crack the code of seriousness on the starting line. He wears his wife's knit black-wool cap. He is also the only elite male wearing a gray short-sleeved T-shirt under his chartreuse singlet, adopting the look of Patrick Ewing's Georgetown teams of the 1980s. Ramaala's appearance is the first clue that he is a bit of a throwback, an earnest iconoclast.

"I'm the laziest guy I know," he said one evening, sitting in his house in Johannesburg a month before the New York City Marathon.

Of course, he had said this after running seventy-five minutes that afternoon with his training group and after staying up all night traveling back to South Africa from a half-marathon in England.

If he were "lazy," then Ramaala, now 35 years old, would only be confirming what his father, Frans, thought of him when he was growing up in the northern mountain village of GaMolepo. "My father never liked my character," Ramaala said.

When he was young, his father, who owned a general store in the village, stressed the importance of working fast. But Ramaala never wanted to rush or to perform even the smallest job quickly; he preferred to be methodical.

When Ramaala told his father he wanted to become a professional runner, Frans was incredulous. "He says, 'You are too slow! You? A runner? Yeah, me too.'" Ramaala laughed at his own imitation and shook his head.

"Problem is," Ramaala added, "with doing things fast, you can't do it right."

When he is not running, Ramaala walks slowly and speaks slowly, but always directly, the closest he comes to putting his law degree to practice. His strength from a deliberate way of life fuels his speed while running.

Ramaala runs to defy his doubters and to honor the country he loves. He runs because the more purposefully he strides, the more real the world beneath his feet becomes.

Other people tried to tell him his place in their world. The white family that employed his mother as a housekeeper during apartheid said he would not make anything of himself, because he was black. His own family initially said he would have more success as a lawyer. Other professional runners said he was crazy not to get a coach; crazy to stick with the marathon, which he never seemed to master as he had the 10 kilometer and half-marathon distances. They said he could not possibly train for marathons in a municipal park running only in a 3.5 kilometer loop.

Traditional South African society said nothing but raised an eyebrow when he chose a white woman, Rodica Moroianu, a runner who was a native of Romania, to be his life partner and started a family with her. The running community in South Africa respects him but wonders when he will run Comrades, the overwhelmingly popular 56-mile ultramarathon that defines distance running in the country.

To all these critics and cynics, Hendrick Ramaala responds with a shrug of his shoulders and a wry grin beneath his mustache. He knows he is different and does not care. He has made peace with his paradox.

Ramaala always possessed a personality distinct from his brothers', who were more impulsive and fiery, prone to getting into fights. "Compared to everyone, he's very different. He has patience. He also has the tenacity," his older brother Legkau said one afternoon when he went to the University of Witwatersrand in Johannesburg, to watch the end of Ramaala's track workout.

Ramaala, the third oldest child in his family, was contemplative like his mother, Sarah. She had much to do every day from before sunrise to 9 p.m., feeding eight children, gathering wood, collecting water, washing clothes, making meals, cleaning the five-bedroom house. She did it slowly, efficiently and without complaint.

While his mother became his confidante, his father wanted Ramaala to work more, at home and at the store. Ramaala walked one hour to and from his missionary school every day and protested that he had no free time because he had to study. "I wanted to be the best at school," Ramaala said. "I wanted to pass well. The father doesn't understand that the school is more important."

Ramaala wanted to be clear on one matter.

"To cut a long story short," he said, "me and the family, we are very, very close. My father is my best friend. When I was younger, me and him, we didn't agree on many things. He was winning, because I was in his house. It was better to keep quiet. I tell the mother sometimes."

When he applied for an academic scholarship to Johannesburg's prestigious University of Witwatersrand in 1989, the mail from his village did not get to the school before the deadline, so he had to reapply, waiting an extra year to matriculate. His mother had already left the family's northern village to work for the English family in Johannesburg. She was five hours away by bus when Ramaala, a teenager, became the manager of the household, cooking for his younger siblings and doling out portions according to age.

The family insisted Sarah work more than 14 hours a day; she could not protest because her own family needed the money. "She was very unlucky, that is all I can say," Ramaala said, shaking his head.

When Ramaala spoke to the English matriarch who hired his mother, "me and the woman, we clashed," he said with a short nod, not wanting to elaborate.

This was in 1990, before the South African government had abolished apartheid. The white children reminded Ramaala of his subservience. "I was never going to be equal to those kids. There was no way," Ramaala said. "It was in their face. The white boys and girls were always going to get the best job. Even if I had the same education, it wasn't going to happen that we would be on top, and we all knew it. And some of them will remind you, 'You can't be above me. You won't be above me.' Which was sad.

"Some didn't want to accept it, even now, that the other people could be on top. They see me, successful. They question, 'How did they get the money?' But we never put a question mark on them. 'Oh, nice car.' Oh, sure, worked hard. But when it's a black guy? Ohhh."

When Ramaala matriculated at Witwatersrand (the city's largest university, with a student body of about 17,500), he tried out for the soccer team. Growing up, the Ramaala boys would form their own team, Ramaala playing left wing and scoring the majority of the goals. On the university level, though, he was too slight to make the team—standing 5 foot 7 and weighing only 125 pounds. Once he was cut, Ramaala drifted to the all-grass track, and he joined the university's track team to stay in shape.

In December 1992, Ramaala ran a 5,000 meter race that is still his most memorable. Why? Because he ran so slowly—15 minutes, 4 seconds, nearly three minutes below the world record pace. That race showed Ramaala how hard he would have to train. "You got to start somewhere," he said.

By 1993, he had shaved his time to 14:36. He graduated with his undergraduate degree in 1994 and continued with his law school studies while continuing to train. In February 1995, he ran 13:24. In 1996, Ramaala completed his law degree and received two job offers to practice, while his older brother, Legkau, who was in law school at the same time with him, did not have any. In the still unsettled post-apartheid economy, Legkau encouraged his younger brother to consider his good fortune and quit running.

"I was disappointed. I wanted him to have a career and get money for the family," said Legkau, who now works long hours as a criminal attorney.

But Ramaala assured them he would soon be able to support them in his own way. His family's reaction changed over the next three years when Ramaala started delivering results, winning a national title in the half-marathon in 1997 and then becoming the world silver medalist at the distance in 1998 and 1999.

"When I saw him perform," Legkau said, "I thought, 'This is his calling.'"

Hendrick and Rodica live in a modest house in the Parktown North section of Johannesburg, an upper-middle-class neighborhood with lush, flowering trees and self-contained villas. The house is up the street from the one-bedroom apartment they lived in for six years. And the house is two blocks from the family home where Ramaala's mother used to work. He grew up in a village without electricity. Not a day goes by that Ramaala is not reminded of his upward path.

The house comes with a pool, a laughable extravagance to him. But his seven-year-old waterbug of a son, Alex, loves it. So Ramaala cleans the pool daily even though he himself does not swim. The pool must be checked for chlorine levels, the floral detritus of the South African spring skimmed off the top.

It is then that the rose bushes bloom magenta around the pool, and the trees flower with purple blooms, tickling the electric fence that separates Ramaala's house from his neighbors'. He and Rodica have lived in the four-bedroom house for a year, and it is still sparse, giving Alex plenty of room to sprint back and forth over the wooden floors when he's not parked in front of the flat-screen television watching the Disney Channel.

They live behind high walls, two electronically controlled gates, and together with their neighbors they pay for an armed security guard to patrol the street. This precaution is normal, even in the better neighborhoods of crime-ridden Johannesburg. Carjackings, robberies and kidnappings are common problems in the city. The province of Gauteng, in which Johannesburg is the largest city, experienced 3,892 carjackings from April to September 2007, according to a public report by the South African police. There were also 3,568 robberies during that time.

Johannesburg was rocked by the senseless death of reggae star Lucky Dube, who was shot to death in front of his teenage son during an attempted carjacking in October 2007. Then in March 2008, the violence would come far closer to home for Ramaala, when men scaled the walls of a house down the block from his and fatally shot an architect inside, also wounding his wife and son, without even attempting robbery.

Ramaala says he does not live in fear, but he is constantly vigilant about safety and maintains a low profile. Ramaala drives a 1992 sky blue Nissan truck and looks both ways before entering his driveway—"that is where the majority of the robberies happen," he said—to make sure that no one follows him in on his bumper. He has an outer gate and an inner gate.

"You get big security, you get a big safe," Ramaala said, adding jokingly: "You buy a rifle like the Texas guys, you buy short guns."

He says the barbed wire and walls that most owners on the block have erected in the last ten years are sadly resonant of another era. Ramaala explains it as an extension of the *laager* mentality, harking back to the nineteenth century when the white English settlers literally circled their wagons to close themselves off against attacks from the Africans. Figuratively, the word *laager* implies an insular, defensive attitude.

Ramaala is a keen social commentator on the problems of post-apartheid South Africa, from government corruption to unemployment. As a student, Ramaala stood in marches of 100,000 people, rallying against apartheid. He was reluctant to be caught in any violence, though, and stayed away from certain rallies. The end of apartheid, while celebrated universally brought other problems locally.

"The motto was Equal Opportunities to All, freedom and whatever. 'South Africa belongs to all,'" Ramaala said, quoting from the preamble to the 1996 South African Constitution, which goes on to say the country is united in its diversity.

"But if you tell the man in the street, 'South Africa is going to enjoy the wealth of the country.' But how?"

Ramaala talks of a disconcerting feeling of entitlement in the black community, people thinking that just because they endured apartheid, they were owed something. This contributes to a culture of laziness, he believes, something he cannot abide.

"People expected too much," he said of the post-apartheid era. "When transition happened, we were all not going to be rich. We were still going to have to work hard. We were going to get an opportunity, if we were lucky."

Ramaala staunchly believes in working to change one's life and respects those who make an honest effort. "I made it happen," he added. "I was one of the lucky ones."

He was also one of the talented ones, blessed with natural speed and determination, but hindered at times by his own stubbornness. After he graduated from law school, he coached himself. He set South African records in the 10K race on the roads and the 10,000-meter race on the track (running 27:29:94 in 1999). Because of his success in the half-marathon, people thought that he could make an easy transition to the full marathon.

Ramaala's first race at that distance proved to be an inauspicious beginning. At the 1999 Chicago Marathon, he was not prepared for temperatures that hovered around the freezing mark. Despite warnings from his agent, John Bicourt (a former Olympian in the steeplechase for Great Britain), Ramaala thought he would be fine wearing only a tank top. He wasn't. He had to drop out midway through the race.

During the next three years, Ramaala could not seem to break through, never placing higher than fifth in major city marathons. His first victory came in near obscurity, in Mumbai, India, in February 2004.

Ramaala was supremely confident leading up to the Athens Olympics in August 2004. But, while committing the fatal flaw of wearing an untested pair of running shoes (he said Nike did not send the pair on time), he also started too fast. In the summer heat of Athens, Ramaala dropped out with a hamstring pull, earning intense criticism from the South African media.

The New York City Marathon had already filled its professional athlete spots by the time his agent appealed to the elite athlete coordinator, David Monti, to take Ramaala. With a New York résumé of fourteenth place in 2002 and fifth in 2001, Ramaala had not exactly made a winning impression.

"Look, he's just not a good marathon runner," Monti told Bicourt. "It's not fair for him to come and get blown away."

But Bicourt insisted that this year would be different. Ramaala believed it, too.

Monti and Mary Wittenberg, the Road Runners' vice president, listened, offering Ramaala no money up front, but paying for his accommodations and negotiating generous bonuses if Ramaala were to finish first, second or third.

His trip to New York got off to a rough start. Ramaala sat in coach (as he always does), and, as usual, did not sleep a minute during his 18-hour flight. Ramaala felt forgotten after he landed at John F. Kennedy Airport. A transportation snafu stranded him and the South African wheelchair racer Ernst Van Dyk at the airport for three hours. When Ramaala finally reached his Manhattan hotel, his room had been given away. Monti, though, found him a room at a smaller hotel down the block, which suited Ramaala perfectly. He slept soundly the first night and was well prepared for Sunday.

The day before the race, Ramaala was walking around the main athletes' hotel when other runners' agents came up to him and said: "Why are you running this? You?"

Ramaala smiled and said little. He quieted the critics the next day by winning in 2:09:28.

"Once I won in 2004, it gave me what I always wanted," Ramaala said. "If you don't win, people doubt you. This proved I was doing the right thing; I can be one of those guys."

When Ramaala returned victorious to Johannesburg, he made sure he immediately thanked his training partners. He threw them a barbecue in the park where they run and brought back New York City Marathon shirts emblazoned with the sunrise over the Verrazano-Narrows Bridge. Three years later, one of the group's least competitive runners, 37-year-old Isaac Masilela, still comes to practice wearing that gift, often days in a row. Ramaala's legacy does not fade.

Today, Ramaala is running the twenty-first marathon of his career. He is in the pack of fifteen elite men charging up the bridge, flanked by an imposing field of three other former winners: Brazil's Marilson Gomes dos Santos (2006), Kenya's Martin Lel (2003) and Rodgers Rop (2002). At 37, the 2004 Olympic champion from Italy, Stefano Baldini, is the oldest of this top group.

If the lead pack were to turn around and glance at the roadway to their left, the runners would witness an onslaught of humanity. They might also witness men emptying their bladders in a steady stream off the side of the bridge. Green bib runners on the lower deck beware.

But Ramaala and his fellow competitors storm off the ramp of the bridge, having already traversed 1.8 miles, unaware of anyone or anything but their pounding hearts.

As he enters the streets of Bay Ridge, Brooklyn, with neat row houses and fans shaking cowbells, Ramaala rushes into the sanctuary that is his world. There is a slight headwind, but nothing overpowering. He has faced far more resistance before.

5

SOLE SEARCHING

Miles 4 and 5, Fourth Avenue, Brooklyn

G od is everywhere on Fourth Avenue.
　　Churches, synagogues, and mosques line both sides of the broad island-divided street, from Pentecostal storefronts to Roman Catholic towers, their names written in Spanish, English and Arabic. This four-mile stretch becomes a stirring advertisement for the unity of faith.

The banner "Marathon of Prayer" hangs on a fence at the corner of Fourth and Ovington avenues, outside the Bay Ridge United Methodist Church, which houses an English-speaking congregation and two others for Korean and Lithuanian members. A band playing steel drums sets up on the grassy front lawn following the ecumenical breakfast.

As much as the New York City Marathon is about the physical experience, it also provides for many a spiritual component. Runners conduct private conversations during the race with themselves, their bodies and their God. In turn, the runners inspire the worshippers who spill onto the street. Devotion, sacrifice, conviction and self-discovery—these essential components of running and religion are not so distinct.

Father Francisco Rodriguez understands this connection as he stands at the corner of Fourth Avenue and 56th Street, cheering the thousands of runners alongside his congregants from La Iglesia Episcopal de San Andres (St. Andrews Episcopal Church).

"Watch the runners," Rodriguez says, "and in the face of the people, you look at God."

This is only Mile 5, he is reminded. At Mile 23, perhaps God might look a little worse for wear. He laughs (he is not a runner) and presses on with his theme: "Runners are not doing this to win, but to finish. They are serving a higher purpose on this day."

The churches and synagogues reflect the individual neighborhoods' immigration patterns; Rodriguez's church is growing, continually adding Mexican, Central American, Ecuadorian and Colombian parishioners. Rodriguez is Cuban. Marathon Sunday reminds him of his own journey, one of struggle and epiphany.

Rodriguez grew up in Cuba and earned his university degree in electrical engineering, but he always felt drawn to the church. He attended a seminary in Matanzas, Cuba, then traveled as a missionary in Central America, the Caribbean and the United States. He returned to Cuba and began working as a chemical engineer in the sugar cane industry and soon felt his employers were discriminating against him. He was not promoted, but his non-Christian co-workers were.

To pursue his true calling, Rodriguez knew he had to leave Cuba. He went first to Miami and then decided to go to New York to attend the General Theological Seminary of the Episcopal Church. He was ordained in 2004. Rodriguez's first congregation was in Sunnyside, Queens, and he supplemented his income by working at a local International House of Pancakes. Later that year, he was appointed to St. Andrews in Brooklyn, to reinvigorate a congregation in need of leadership. His small church in Sunset Park, with white walls and dark-stained wooden beams, is open to anyone. "I want to bring hope to the people," he says.

And after watching the masses in sneakers stream past on this Sunday, Rodriguez brings the Marathon to the pulpit. His sermon?

"The Marathon," he says, "shows to us love, hope, unity, joy, solidarity, companionship—like the gospel of God."

Fans four deep line both sides of Fourth Avenue as they stand clapping and shouting, some banging on pots and pans for extra emphasis. Some families sit together on folding lawn chairs to watch the parade of runners pass them, as if it were the Fourth of July. One man stands nearby selling cotton candy. The party is in full swing.

By the time Pam Rickard enters the religious straightaway of Fourth Avenue, she has hit her rhythm, buoyed by her strong legs and her Christian faith. She wears a special white T-shirt, on which she has painted in red the words to her favorite hymn: "It Is Well with My Soul."

The hymn was written in 1873 by Horatio Spafford after he suffered a litany of personal tragedy: He lost his fortune in the Great Chicago Fire of 1871, his son died and then later his four daughters died in a transatlantic boat accident. His wife, who was on the boat, sent back the cable: "Saved Alone."

The hymn speaks of newfound tranquility after hardship, such as Pam has found after years of alcohol abuse. The sentiment stirs others around her.

"Sweet!" a male runner shouts from behind Pam, startling her until she realizes he is referring to her shirt. "Man, that's where we all need to get."

"That's one of my favorite hymns," another man says, "I am going to have that in my head the rest of the race."

Pam needs these reminders wherever she goes; they are sign-posts to her recovery. In her small, four-bedroom house in Rocky Mount, Virginia, Pam hangs index cards on mirrors, on kitchen corkboards, in painting frames, above the computer inscribed with words in black marker:

"Truth. Humility. Patience."

"Remember the illusion, not the reality" is written on the label of an empty gin bottle that sits on her dresser.

At first, she drank only wine, a couple of glasses every night. That's what her mother always used to drink. Then, steadily, Pam started drinking any kind of liquor when she came home from work, and at other odd hours. She began hiding bottles in linen closets and behind shampoo bottles.

Once, to fool her husband, Tom, who was starting to get anxious about her self-destructive habit, she poured wine into orange juice cartons in the bathroom of the supermarket while Tom waited for her in the car. It was the kind of orange juice (low-calorie) that nobody else in the family would drink. She started ordering cases from Wine of the Month club and found herself making excuses to the FedEx delivery man about upcoming parties. The parties were only for herself.

Perhaps in retrospect, it was only fitting that Pam began her running career with a hangover. The morning after homecoming at Ohio University, Pam's friends had convinced her to run a 5 kilometer race. Having partied and smoked her usual pack of cigarettes the day before, she walked part of the race. But still, she was intrigued.

Pam describes herself as a "couch potato-prima donna" in her high school days in suburban Cleveland. She started running more regularly after that college race as a way of maintaining her weight.

When she discovered she had natural talent, she quit smoking and began getting serious about running.

Pam and Tom both graduated from Ohio University's journalism program in 1984, and he found a job as a reporter for the *Daily Jeffersonian* in Cambridge, Ohio, near the Pennsylvania border, while she worked in advertising for the *Pittsburgh Press*. The couple soon relocated to Virginia, where Pam got a job at the *Roanoke Times* and started winning local distance races in her age group. She threw herself into training for her first marathon, learning one week before the 1988 Cleveland Marathon that she was pregnant with her first child. Pam ran her first marathon anyway, five weeks pregnant—in 4 hours, 12 minutes.

While carrying her daughter Abby, she stopped drinking, as she would throughout each of her three pregnancies. "For some reason, I wasn't able to drink," Pam said in her modest living room in Rocky Mount, two months before the New York City Marathon. "I guess it was just the maternal instinct."

She ran until she was eight months pregnant. She breast-fed Abby for six weeks and started drinking again the day she stopped. Nine months after giving birth ("like Paula Radcliffe," Pam exclaimed, "except I had a C-section!"), she ran the 1989 Columbus Marathon in 4:35, which is still her slowest time of any marathon. Disappointed, Pam trained harder for Columbus in 1990 and finished in 3:31, still her personal best.

She realizes now that her drive to push her body so hard in both running and drinking was motivated by the same thing:

"Fear," she said. "Fear of not living up. I always felt like a little bit of a fraud even though I've always had a lot of success."

Fear of not fulfilling her own impossibly high expectations tormented Pam in her career, her running and her parenting. Lacking the ability to recognize her success and then process genuine satisfaction from her accomplishments, she turned to alcohol to relieve her anxiety.

"What's really the catch–22 with that, she would work harder and she would be successful, and people would say, 'Great job,'" Tom said. "And then she would be afraid that she wouldn't be able to maintain that. The next time wouldn't be as good. That fear would never let go."

Pam began exercising harder and longer, intent on winning local races, as if to outrun her disease. "She wanted to have it all," Tom said. "The fact that she was running allowed her body not to break down as quickly."

Pam admits that her fear and addictive behavior have familial roots. Her parents divorced when she was 13. Although she is careful not to blame her father, she describes him as an inveterate liar, a man who stuttered but exploited his disadvantage for sympathy in business deals. Pam described her mother as quite the opposite, "genuine and extraordinary." Both of her parents' fathers struggled with alcoholism, Pam said, and her maternal grandfather committed suicide, likely as a result.

Pam was becoming estranged from her children and her husband, who had identified her wildly erratic behavior as a problem but not yet an addiction.

"We couldn't understand why Mom couldn't just STOP," Abby recalled in an e-mail, the way she said she was most comfortable communicating. "I felt hurt and betrayed and totally disgusted with her, and it was at its utmost when no one was doing anything about it. There seemed to be no end in sight, and no one was stepping up and calling it out to be WRONG and not normal motherly behavior."

Abby, who dislikes running, said she had resented—no, "truly hated"—her mother since she had been in middle school. Pam's running only fueled her daughter's resentment. "I always felt that she used it as a crutch," Abby said, "not only to make herself feel better, but to win praise and validation from others in her frightfully unstable world."

That world was consuming Pam's life, so much that she even stopped running after she gave birth to Sophie in 2003.

"I look back on it now and realize how much I enabled," Tom said. "There were nights when Pam would have blackouts, not the unconscious kind, but when she would walk around and not remember a thing."

Tom is an elementary school librarian, patient, loving and religious, not the angry type. But even he admitted to getting frustrated when he would come home after Pam returned from her job as a fundraiser for the Roanoke YMCA and see her already drunk.

"I was pretty pissed off," he said softly.

"When it started to get really bad, I started looking for it. I said, 'If I get rid of it, she'll be OK tonight.' It really got to the point, each night, where it was, 'What's tonight going to be like? Will we have a good night?'

"It got to the point where there were no good nights."

"There were times," Abby recalled, "when I truly hoped this addiction would kill her."

Pam was arrested for driving under the influence in November 2004. In March 2005, she was arrested a second time for DUI on the way home from visiting a donor to the new YMCA building in Roanoke. For that offense, she was sentenced to 10 days in the Roanoke City Jail, an experience that was horrifying, but not frightful enough to derail her drinking.

When she was released, the court ordered Pam to have an interlocking machine installed in her car to monitor her drinking; she had to blow into the breathalyzer and be clean in order for the car to start. She cheated on February 4, 2006, when she took Abby's car to the local convenience store for more alcohol. Pam was stopped by the police in the parking lot, looking tired and disoriented in the car. It was her third DUI arrest.

"Any one of her three DUIs could have resulted in a death, her death or the death of other people," Tom said. "It didn't. She just got pulled over."

Tom organized a family intervention in February 2006 when everyone was gathered for the wake for his brother-in-law, Jimmy. Pam, who was drunk, was spouting off about her third DUI arrest. Eventually her family convinced Pam that she needed treatment, but it took another month to get her there.

"I just love her like crazy," Tom said. "I'd get angry at her, scared, but unless I'm just fooling myself, I never considered leaving. I knew that our family was supposed to stay together. I knew that she had to stop drinking."

On April 17, 2006, Pam had her last drink and entered the treatment facility in Williamsburg, Virginia. Insurance would pay only $503 of the $15,000 fee. Pam and Tom were stuck, so they allowed her father to foot the bill. They took out a $25,000 home equity loan to pay him back.

Pam spent one month away from her family at the Williamsburg Place treatment facility. She stopped drinking, though she took up smoking again and started to surrender her will to the Alcoholics Anonymous program. She returned to Rocky Mount in May and attended ninety meetings in ninety days with AA. Meanwhile, sentencing for her third DUI arrest would be delayed by bureaucracy until September.

At her sentencing hearing on September 28, 2006, the Franklin Circuit Court judge, William N. Alexander II, wanted Pam to understand the severity of her actions. Her friends and boss testified as character witnesses in hopes she would receive a more lenient jail term, or none at all.

Judge Alexander had heard enough.

"I'm sick to death of it," Alexander said as he reprimanded her and the entire courtroom, Pam recalled. "You think you can get away with it, and you can't get away with it. You're going. Right now."

Judge Alexander sentenced her to ninety days and a year's probation following her jail term and fined her $2,500. The judge allowed her to go home, say good-bye to her children and return that evening to jail. Rachel, then 11, had just gotten home from school. She was dazed. Abby, at 17, was furious and heartbroken. She could not forget what her mother told her three-year-old sister, Sophie.

"I need you to remember two things," Pam said, as she knelt down to talk to Sophie. "One, I love you. And two, I'm coming home."

With her mother incarcerated, Abby said she tried to make life as normal as possible for her sisters. She and her father became the carpooling service, while they all shared the cooking, the cleaning and the laundry.

"The things moms usually do, we had to do," Rachel recalled in September 2007, when her mother was not in the house. She spoke with more than a trace of teenage resentment. "I learned independence earlier than I had to. I was angry because of Sophie," Rachel added. Every day, Sophie would ask when her mother would be returning. They told her she was in a hospital getting well.

"I look back on that time last year," Tom said, "and I think, 'Man, how did we get through that?' You just do."

In jail, Pam would wonder the same.

Now she makes her way amid the multitudes, trying not to trip over the runners around her while maintaining a steady

8-minute, 40-second pace. Today, Pam feels swept up in the race's flow like a fish in a school.

She passes five-story tenements, bodegas, liquor stores, Chinese and Mexican restaurants and laundromats, all interspersed with various places of worship. She does not bother to look down the side streets stacked with pale brick two-story row houses built nearly a century ago. Mile Marker 5, on the corner of Fourth Avenue and 42nd Street, is but one avenue away from the namesake of the neighborhood, Sunset Park. The 24.5-acre park, stretching from Fifth Avenue to Seventh, affords some of the best panoramas of Brooklyn and Manhattan. From here, someone might have glimpsed Pam's near miss and witnessed the uplifting communal strength of the Marathon.

As Pam veers in toward a water station, she tries to slow down long enough to grab a cup, only she feels the force of the runners pushing her from behind her. The momentum sends her sprawling awkwardly toward the table, almost to certain injury. In that instant of instability, she thinks, "Well, here I go. This could be bad." Pam wonders whether she could recover to run the next twenty miles, until a female runner suddenly grabs her white "It Is Well with My Soul" shirt and pulls her back away from the table.

"I'm so sorry. Thank you!" Pam calls to the woman.

"Don't worry about it! No problem," the woman responds as Pam's heart races with adrenaline and she continues on her way.

During her training in the foothills of the Blue Ridge Mountains, Pam found comfort in her long, solitary runs where she could manage every movement. Coming to New York, Pam knew that no matter how prepared she felt, she would not be able to control every variable on the course, from potholes to congestion.

"I put myself in the hands of the Marathon," she will say.

Those were the hands that kept her from falling.

The elite women have no crowds to battle, no concerns about how and when to stop for water. Their bottles are specially marked—the athletes prepared them the day before—and waiting on designated tables throughout the course. Just past 78th Street, still on Fourth Avenue, Paula Radcliffe grabs her cotton candy pink plastic bottle with the curvy straw from the table and sips the energy replacement liquid before tossing it to the curb. Gete Wami has picked up her bottle easily from the table and soon discards it as well. A silent, symbiotic companionship is starting to emerge on the Brooklyn streets between the pair.

Wami knew Radcliffe had the fastest résumé in the field today, but she did not expect her to go out quite this fast—Radcliffe ran the second mile, downhill off the bridge and into Brooklyn, in 4:59.

I am just going to have to stay with her, Wami tells herself. She is the only one who does.

By the time they hit Mile Marker 3, Radcliffe is one full step ahead of Wami, striking a pose that will become the postcard of the day. Together, the pair passes through Bay Ridge and Leif Ericson Park in the former Scandinavian, Irish and Italian neighborhood—now also populated by immigrants from the Middle East and Russia. At that point, both women held a 7-second lead over Jelena Prokopcuka.

The race's defending champion decided after the first mile to run at her own pace, forming a second pack with the reigning Boston Marathon champion, Lidiya Grigoryeva, and world champion Catherine Ndereba. By Mile Marker 4, however, Radcliffe and Wami's lead has already increased exponentially to 17 seconds. Approaching Mile Marker 5 on median-divided Fourth Avenue, the lead pair zooms to 28 seconds ahead. More than four blocks behind, Prokopcuka tries not to think about the race that is quickly getting away from her. To catch Radcliffe and Wami now would be a foolish expenditure of energy. She tells herself to stick to the pace she knows she can maintain, to focus on leg turnover and relax the body. There are still plenty of miles left to run.

6

EXTRA LETTER, EXTRA HELP

Mile 6, Fourth Avenue, Sunset Park, Brooklyn

Harrie Bakst is crying. He has been crying actually during each of the previous five miles—on the bridge, through Bay Ridge and now in Sunset Park. Harrie waves to fans and high-fives children lining the street, passing block after block of churches, storefronts and schools, some with Arabic writing.

"You have Muslim people sitting there and I'm the Jewish guy and I'm slapping them on the hand," Harrie will say.

For many runners, the support today extends from the anonymous sidewalk fans, to the volunteers working the water stops, to family and friends stationed along the route. Rich Bakst is running on Harrie's right shoulder and is more excited for his brother than for himself. Rich gives Harrie the position closer to the curb, so he can be nearer to the fans reading his T-shirt and calling out his name. Rich wants Harrie to have the glory, to feel what he felt the year before. So much has happened in one year.

"Go, Harrie! You can do it, Harrie!" the fans call even though they do not know him.

And that's when it kicks in—when Harrie processes everything that has happened to him since February. In the middle of Brooklyn's largest thoroughfare, with the sun shining and his brother by his side, he feels alive. "I'm running a freakin' marathon," Harrie thinks with equal parts defiance and gratitude.

Harrie" is not a common spelling for a boy's name. His mother, Ellen, explained why she chose it. Her father was named Harry Solomon and he died at age 78, when Ellen was pregnant with her second son. In the Jewish tradition, she named him after a departed relative, but decided to give her son an extra letter.

"For life," Ellen said.

On a chilly mid-December Sunday in 2006, that extra letter did not energize Harrie at all when he found himself walking the last few miles of the Joe Kleinerman 10K run in Central Park. He was unable to keep pace with Rich. Harrie did not particularly enjoy distance running and did not think he was good at it; he had played varsity football and baseball at his private high school, Riverdale Country School, in the Bronx.

But Harrie was at that race to run for Rich, who was already planning to train for his second New York City Marathon. The brothers had mostly played stickball as kids. Neither ran for sport or fun.

"Running in the Bronx was all you did when someone was chasing you for money," Harrie recalled a few weeks before the Marathon. He was mugged, he added, as a seventh grader.

Rich gravitated toward running when he was in college and medical school, since it fit his more analytical, introverted personality. Harrie had the opposite personality—impulsive and extroverted. Despite their differences and the three years separating them, they had always been close. They shared a room growing up in their Riverdale apartment, and during their final years at New York University, they lived together in a one-bedroom apartment in the Murray Hill neighborhood of Manhattan.

Rich was finishing his fourth year of medical school at NYU while Harrie was a senior there, applying to law schools and thinking about creating a consulting business in sports philanthropy. He was the president of NYU's Sports Business Society and planned to be part of a trip to Johannesburg over the 2007 spring break to study the economic and social impact of the 2010 World Cup on the city. Rich had arranged for Harrie to see his doctor for the necessary immunizations in early February, one week after his twenty-second birthday.

During that appointment, Rich's primary care doctor was concerned when he felt something in Harrie's neck that Harrie himself had never felt. That doctor referred Harrie to an ear, nose and throat specialist. Upon examining Harrie, and to Harrie's utter horror, the specialist blurted out the three words no one ever wants to hear from a doctor: "Oh my God!"

Harrie swallowed his anger and fear. The biopsy confirmed a malignant tumor on his salivary gland; it was adenoid cystic carcinoma, a rare form of cancer, especially in a 22-year-old. "My whole life turned upside down," Harrie said.

Rich was determined to steady his brother's life. He sprang into action the day of the diagnosis, picking up Harrie's medical slides and marching his brother uptown to Memorial Sloan-Kettering Cancer Center, where Rich had recently interviewed for an internship. Rich secured an appointment with Dr. Jatin Shah, chief of the Head and Neck Service in the hospital's surgery department. Shah told Harrie not to jump to too many conclusions; they would know more after surgery.

Escorting Harrie to the operating room, Rich was the last person to talk to his brother before the surgery on March 21, 2007. Their parents, Ellen and Larry, stood tearfully in the waiting room. After the surgery, Shah told Harrie that he had removed a lump the size of a fig as well as 13 lymph nodes. The cancer, according to Harrie, had been in an intermediary stage—neither early nor advanced, but this was still not particularly good news. "South Africa saved my life," Harrie said. "No joke."

The surgery was on a Wednesday, and Harrie had a human resources exam at NYU on Monday. He checked himself out of the hospital after one day and aced the exam. "I was like a freak patient," Harrie said. "Yeah, my neck was stiff, but I felt amazing."

He felt relieved, as if the hardest part of having cancer was over; at least, that is what Rich told him. Harrie knew he would need radiation treatments, but he blamed Rich for not preparing him when he was told two weeks after the surgery about the side effects—extreme fatigue, loss of hair, loss of taste buds and terrible throat sores.

To a college senior who had seemed perfectly healthy only a month earlier, the sudden puncture in Harrie's invincibility was even more jarring than the diagnosis. He was furious. In a fog, Harrie took a phone call in the cab that was from a potential first client for his sports philanthropy business: the vice president of a coffee company in Tanzania that is owned by Jackie Robinson's son, David. In a moment of despairing uncertainty, Harrie decided to use his pain as an impetus to help others.

"I saw cancer as an opportunity," Harrie said. "The key to business and life is to find value in everything."

Every morning, he and Rich took a taxi from their Murray Hill apartment on 32nd Street, going 35 blocks up First Avenue for Harrie's 7:45 radiation appointment on the fourth floor of Memorial Sloan-Kettering. In the beginning, Harrie would dash home and then go across town to NYU. By the third week, however, the side effects had intensified, and Harrie had barely enough energy to get to class.

He felt worse when he googled survival rates for his rare type of cancer. The statistics were chilling. One study he found said that if a patient survived five years without a recurrence, then the survival rate was 89 percent. Another study showed that patients who lived 15 years after the initial cancer detection only had a 40 percent survival rate.

Harrie had to do something to outpace his uncertain future. At his gym, he started running three miles on a treadmill three times a week during off-hours because he was self-conscious about his appearance. His hair had started to fall out in the back of his head, near his ears. His scar was still red and raw. He felt debilitated.

"It got worse, and I kept doing it. I don't know if it was to prove to myself that I could, but it helped mentally," he said of his running. "It was not only to clear my head, but to get away from the stuff that I was consuming on the Internet.

"It was also like, 'All right, I have cancer. So what!'"

In his fifth week of radiation, on May 22, 2007, Harrie completed the 3 mile Wall Street Run with his brother. One section of the back of his head was bald, and his throat burned so much he felt as though he were swallowing nails. He started crying at Mile 1, overjoyed to be moving. At the end of the race, his mouth and nose were so dry, he started bleeding.

"I have blood on my shirt and people are like, 'What the hell happened to this kid?'" he recalled.

The kid had become a runner.

Harrie and Rich slow down to a walk at the water stop between 23rd and 24th streets on Fourth Avenue, as their Fred's Team coach, Jeff Rochford, taught them to do. They pinch the cup, so as not to spill the water, and take a brief break.

Today in the Sunset Park neighborhood of Brooklyn, however, there is one man who never stops running.

"From 23rd Street to 24th Street," Carmine Santoli says.

At eighty-one, Santoli oversees his own empire on Marathon Sunday, just on that one Sunset Park block of brick tenements and storefronts. This is Santoli's 27th New York City Marathon as captain of the Mile 6 aid station, and he has seen everything in his changing neighborhood.

What was once Italian, Irish, Polish and Finnish, is now increasingly populated by Latin American immigrants, as well as Pakistani, Indian and Chinese. One landmark has stayed virtually the same for more than 150 years—the 478-acre Green-Wood Cemetery is the neighborhood's centerpiece, stretching east from Fifth Avenue past 10th Avenue, and north from 36th Street to 20th Street. New York luminaries, including Leonard Bernstein, Horace Greeley and Charles Ebbets, are among the half million souls interred here. Santoli has no plans to join them any time soon.

Over the years, his gray hair has grown wispy, and he has shrunk inside the old oversize Marathon jacket. But it is Santoli's lucky jacket, and he would not dream of updating it. Fred Lebow gave it to him personally. Santoli gives out the new T-shirts and ponchos and hats to the other 200 volunteers, friends, family members and schoolchildren who help him.

The day actually began at midnight, when the Marathon organizers dropped off seventy-two tables. Santoli went back to sleep until 4 a.m., when the shipment of water and Gatorade arrived. Santoli's first thought was to make sure people would not steal the supplies. Early in the morning, he saw a man who must have been close to 70 years old walk off with two cases of water, holding six jugs each. *Walk* might be too strong a word. The man hobbled, sweating profusely, and shoved the cases into his car. When Santoli confronted the man, he denied it. Santoli was too busy to harangue the petty thief or explain to the policemen on the corner what happened. This type of thing happens every year.

Santoli patrols his block the best he can. He is one of 10,000 Marathon volunteers today, an army on virtually every corner of the course, doing every job imaginable for only a T-shirt, a poncho, a hat and a story or two. Many neighborhood volunteers have been on their corners just as long as Santoli, making the Marathon their social event of the year. For the faithful New York Road Runners volunteers who bond as they work to organize smaller local races over decades, the New York City Marathon becomes even more special.

For Santoli, this is a day of celebration. His two granddaughters and two great-grandsons come to volunteer. Five friends take the day off from their Costco jobs just to work on the block. One volunteer, a nurse, has come for the last 25 years. Santoli has food for 20 in his apartment—thanks to a six-foot-long sandwich he ordered.

"I have kids that were eight and 10 years old when they started. Now they're grown men, they have families and they bring them down, too," Santoli says. "People from New Jersey, Connecticut, they wait for this day—it's a get-together.

"I look forward to it. I really do," he adds. "I see so many of my old friends. I see where I can help a person in a wheelchair. I see an old woman, must be 85 years old, walking. It makes you feel good that you can help someone."

Of course, not everyone wants to be helped. Santoli is approached by a group of older Polish women demanding to cross the street to attend church at Our Lady of Czestochowa. There are 30,000 runners rushing past between 10:30 a.m. and 11:30 a.m., just when Mass begins.

"I can't allow these women who are 80, 90 years old to cross the street. The runners will knock 'em down," Santoli says. He tells them to take the subway one stop, cross under the station and then take it back one stop. The women do not listen, instead turning around and going up to St. John the Evangelist at Fifth Avenue and 21st Street.

By 8 a.m., the volunteers have stirred the powdered Gatorade mix with water. They have poured Gatorade and water into cups, stacked three tiers high, 200 cups in each tier, according to Marathon protocol. Once the inspector from the Road Runners leaves, however, Santoli instructs his volunteers to stack the cups in five tiers, separated by cardboard. "If you do it only three tiers, the water will all be gone," he explains. He will prepare 57,000 cups of water and Gatorade today.

"When the first group comes, it's beautiful," he says. "Half an hour later, people are just running over you."

His wife, Ann, is standing in their second-floor apartment, which overlooks the street. She shouts to Santoli to get inside, fearful he will be crushed.

"It's too many people," Santoli admits. His aid station operates on both the east and west sides of the street and also has nine tables set up on the avenue's median to accommodate the mass of runners. "When they come down, it's like a whole load of horses coming at you."

For forty years, he stayed out of life's fray, fixing radiators in cranes above the Brooklyn piers, some fifteen stories high. Santoli's hands are large and leathery from the job, his face wizened and kind from life. His father, Philip, lived to be 92. Santoli is the third youngest in a family of nine siblings.

Santoli and Ann have lived on this corner of Fourth Avenue and 24th Street in their four-bedroom apartment for fifty-six years.

When they moved in, the building had offered low-income housing, and they paid only $52.50 a month. Now the rent is $613 a month, still extraordinarily cheap in this burgeoning Brooklyn market.

The traditional boundaries of Sunset Park stretched from 65th Street north to 17th Street, at the Prospect Expressway. But recently, with the most desirable apartments in nearby Park Slope to the north filling up quickly, the trendy neighborhood has pushed its boundaries south toward Santoli's block. He said his landlord told him an apartment identical to his is now renting at $1,800. The landlord offered $25,000 and three months free rent to move. Santoli laughed. The man might as well have asked him to give up working the Marathon.

This year, even Santoli stops scurrying around when he sees Paula Radcliffe and Gete Wami blur by his block. He is mesmerized by their taut, contrasting bodies and their warp speed.

By Mile 6, Paula Radcliffe and Gete Wami have opened up a 44-second lead over Jelena Prokopcuka, who is running a good four blocks behind in a second pack with Lidiya Grigoryeva and Catherine Ndereba. Radcliffe and Wami run 5:16 for Mile 6, while the second pack trails at 5:26.

Santoli has his back to the course a half-hour later when the dozen runners in the men's pack race by at 5:01 for Mile 6. "When they run," Santoli said, "one step is four of ours."

The leaders are flying in a V formation like a flock of geese heading north. They shift back and forth until Hendrick Ramaala takes the lead, and the others fall in single file behind him. Ramaala is frustrated, his blood boiling in the cool air, his legs yearning to shake up the formation. His mind is racing.

Why isn't anyone pushing the pace? Must I do this myself?

Just after Santoli's water stop, Ramaala answers his own question by breaking into a sprint that is astounding not only for its speed—

a pace of 4:27—but for its timing. Most runners would think this a little early in the race to be expending so much energy. But Ramaala is calculating. At 35, he knows that he runs best if he jump-starts his legs; a languid pace in the first few miles will doom him.

So Ramaala runs a fartlek, a term of Swedish origin that means "speed play." In Swedish, the word has a rather lighthearted connotation—more like "playing around." The concept can be as simple as challenging a training partner to the next traffic light, or it can be part of interval training. It is not usually intended for competition.

But the race has a different tone this year because its director, Mary Wittenberg, has eliminated pacesetters (known as "rabbits") as an experiment to promote champion-style racing.

In the past, rabbits served as escorts, enabling the elite runners to avoid strategizing and run on cruise control until the 16-mile mark, when the rabbit would drop out. The afternoon before a race, elite runners would convene at a technical meeting and decide on the half-marathon split time the rabbit would aim for. In 2006, it was supposed to be 64 minutes but it turned into 65:34, voiding the purpose of the pacesetter.

Ramaala takes it upon himself to play that role today, to stir the lactic acid in his legs a little earlier than usual, and to push the comfort level of the other runners. He is not being altruistic, just realistic.

"I am not going to come in even third in a race like this," he thinks. "I am going to come in way behind."

A fan's sign between Miles 6 and 7 captures the spirit of his sprint. Run Like the Wind, the poster reads.

Ramaala's surges cause the pack to break apart, and some runners fall back, but only temporarily. If nothing else, Ramaala has helped inject some personality into the race and establish a sense of intrigue for the day.

7

SECOND PLACE

Mile 7, Park Slope, Brooklyn

By now, the third, fourth and fifth place women in this race are specks in the distance on Fourth Avenue, a good ten blocks behind Gete Wami, who is one shoestring length behind Paula Radcliffe. With the sun above and a little behind them, they cast two faint silhouettes onto the street in front of them. As Radcliffe and Wami continue to chase their shadows, they cannot elude their shared past.

They are once again a package deal: yin and yang, Mutt and Jeff, expressive and stone-faced, two mothers reprising a rivalry that began when they were teenagers, 16 years and 32 races ago.

Their first race against each other came at the World Junior Cross Country championships in 1991 when Wami finished fifth and Radcliffe fifteenth. The next year at these championships in Boston, with snow blanketing the course, Radcliffe won her first international title and Wami finished ninth.

From that day on, though, Wami would dominate. She won 26 races against Radcliffe on all surfaces—notably on the track and in cross-country. In the five races that they finished first and second,

Wami won four times, but each time by rail-thin margins of one second to four seconds. These two rivals, however, have not competed against each other since 2001 and have never run in the same marathon together—until today.

Although Radcliffe and Wami were both born in December, albeit a year apart, they contrast as much as a running twosome could. Radcliffe towers at nearly 5 foot 8—about eight inches taller than Wami. Radcliffe has a strained face when running, pasty skin, a peacock head bob, a blond ponytail, dark sunglasses and a high, swaying carriage. Wami has a stone face and deep brown skin, a motionless upper body, a wispy ponytail, a white skullcap and a low-slung running style.

When Wami runs, she looks as though she is always leaning into the finish line tape. Radcliffe looks as though she is running up the side of a mountain.

"One thing is characteristic of the Ethiopian girls: They run with such grace and appear effortless; they always look comfortable," Radcliffe wrote in her autobiography, *Paula: My Story So Far*. "I know, however, that this is just an illusion; the ease is more apparent than real. They are hurting, too, it's just that it doesn't show. They can go from looking so comfortable to beaten in a couple of strides. It can be frustrating, because you never know how close you are to breaking them, but it's important to remember how close you *can* be."

The passage prefaced the description of the 1999 International Association of Athletics Federations World Championships at Seville, Spain, where Radcliffe and Wami competed in the 10,000 meters. Wami, after sitting on Radcliffe's shoulder the whole race, surged past her in the final 400 meters. Radcliffe tried to match her burst, but Wami had one more surge left and captured the race by 2.17 seconds.

Two years later, Radcliffe reversed her reputation for getting beaten by Ethiopian women in the eleventh hour. At the 2001 IAAF World Cross Country Championships at Ostend, Belgium, Radcliffe ran with Wami most of the way on the 7.7 kilometer long course. When Wami surged, this time Radcliffe outkicked her for the victory. "No one likes losing," Wami told the media after the race, graciously adding: "But if anyone deserves to win this title, it is Paula. She was great."

The following day, Wami outsprinted Radcliffe for the victory on the 4.1 kilometer short course. Radcliffe was ecstatic that she broke her drought the previous day, but she would keep the short-course defeat in the back of her mind.

She would also remember her last lengthy conversation with Wami when they sat together for drug testing during those championships. They talked about motherhood. Wami told Radcliffe she was eager to get pregnant as soon as possible and start a family; Radcliffe hoped to have a family one day, too, just not yet.

Six years later, Isla, Radcliffe's nine-month-old daughter, is taking her first tentative steps on her own this weekend in New York. Wami's four-year-old, pigtailed daughter, Eva, stayed with relatives back in Addis Ababa.

Were these two mothers to linger in Park Slope, this trendy neighborhood of late-Victorian brownstone row houses and stately homes, they would be right at home among the young parents pushing stylish strollers and running after children in nearby Prospect Park.

Now Wami is too busy chasing after Radcliffe, as they cross over the footprints of history.

From 20th Street to 3rd Street, the course rolls gently downhill, and together the women gather momentum in the final stretch of Fourth Avenue, unaware that British soldiers and American colonists had once trod the same path. A block before the Mile 7 marker, the Old Stone House sits to the right of the course, at 3rd Street. The red roof is visible from the street, even if the original 1699 Dutch farmhouse has been rebuilt. Tucked sideways into a block-long park with handball courts behind a chain-link fence, it is now a museum commemorating the spot where the colonists made a courageous, albeit losing stand in the first major battle of the Revolutionary War.

Later, in 1883, the Old Stone House had a more practical use: as the clubhouse of the team that became the Brooklyn Dodgers.

Yankees and Dodgers, baseball and war—none of this matters today to these two extraordinary female runners. But at some point, one will have to declare independence.

Today Wami is running in second place, a position that is familiar to her, and not in a distasteful way. In Ethiopia, Wami has quietly thrived next to the country's legendary runners, Haile Gebrselassie and Derartu Tulu, who established their fame just as Wami was beginning her career. Gebrselassie, the men's marathon world record holder and multiple track gold medalist, has been an international track and field superstar for 15 years. Tulu became the first black African woman to win an Olympic gold medal, in the 10,000 meters, at the 1992 Barcelona Games.

In a country where women are still trying to break out of their traditionally subservient roles, Tulu, who is five years older than Wami, empowered a new generation of Ethiopian runners. Fatuma Roba won the Olympic gold medal in the marathon at the 1996 Atlanta Games; Wami herself won a bronze medal in the 10,000 meters at Atlanta.

After Tulu gave birth to her daughter, she returned to the Olympic stage at the 2000 Sydney Games and earned another gold medal in the 10,000 meters. Wami won a silver medal, while Radcliffe finished fourth.

"It's true, Gete is a bit in the shadow of Tulu," said Wami's husband and coach, Getaneh Tessema. "But she knows who she is and what she has done."

Wami does not display the medals and trophies she has won at her new house in the hills of Addis Ababa, less than a mile from Gebrselassie's house. She gives some of her prizes to family or friends—per Ethiopian custom—and keeps the others stashed in her dresser drawers.

Her modesty is born of her upbringing and the importance she places on her family. Wami, whose full given name is Getenesh, is just like her mother, Zenevich; they both live for children and not only their own.

Wami grew up in north-central Ethiopia, far from the southern highlands of the Arsi region that spawned the champions Tulu, Gebrselassie and the middle-distance star, Kenenisa Bekele. Her mountainous village of Chacha is about 75 miles northeast of Addis Ababa. Wami was the oldest of six, but her parents' house always seemed to hold more than a dozen children. Every day, Wami's mother would invite neighboring children from the street, for snacks or to play, just to fill the house with laughter.

Wami would help her mother with the farm chores, milking the cows, collecting the eggs from the chickens. When she was 13 and at school, Wami first discovered how much she loved to run. She hid it from her mother and father.

"They thought she was going to learn," Tessema explained. "At the same time, she was learning and running."

Soon they discovered her secret, and they argued with her. This was not acceptable behavior for a girl, they said. The more her parents told her not to run, the more she protested. "But I like to run!" she told them.

It was not until she began to win local races and was offered a spot with the prestigious Omedla sports club that her parents relented. They saw her talent as a means to help the family financially. Wami moved to Addis Ababa at age 17 and was overjoyed to earn her first salary—$14 a month as a runner for the Ethiopian police club, established in 1948. Gebrselassie is the club's most famous member.

In 1990, she met Haile Gebrselassie and Tessema, who was then one of Ethiopia's promising middle-distance runners. Wami won world cross-country titles while training in the capital city, but Tessema fled the country to avoid being conscripted during Ethiopia's bloody border war with Eritrea. A refugee, Tessema settled in the Netherlands, and his running talent got him discovered there by Jos Hermens, a prominent Dutch agent. Soon Tessema started competing in that country.

But on the way to a cross-country competition in rural Holland on December 31, 1996, Tessema's career ended tragically. His life nearly did, too. Tessema was driving himself to the competition when his car broke down. He pulled over to the side of a curved road to open the hood, and, although Tessema was in the emergency lane, an 18-wheeler veered off the curve and struck him. Nearly every bone in his body was broken, and doctors said he would never walk again.

He was in the hospital for a month, and Wami flew immediately to be with him during his arduous rehabilitation. They were married two years later.

"Every day is special; for me it is extra," Tessema said, his eyes welling with tears when he confirmed the story he does not like to tell himself. "It is more than extra to have this life."

When he recovered, Hermens gave him a job in his sports agency. Tessema now serves as a coach and manager of both the men's and women's marathon squads in Ethiopia.

Beneath his permanent smile, Tessema has a devilishly sweet nature. He described how he embarrassed Wami at their wedding, passionately planting a kiss on her lips. That was considered shocking in Ethiopian culture, Tessema explained. Wami, who was next to him at the time, laughed demurely, but she rolled her eyes slightly as if to say, "What am I going to do with you?"

They are a loving couple, showing no signs of the struggles they have endured together. After the Sydney Olympics—when Wami won a silver medal in the 5,000 meters and a bronze in the 10,000 meters—they tried to start a family. It was not easy at first, and Wami visited several fertility doctors. She did not want to take any fertility drugs while training however.

"She always wanted babies, having a family and children, as many as possible—that was her dream," Tessema said.

"That was my only dream," Wami added in Amharic, with her husband translating. "So far, only one! That is the plan—after the Olympics, to have more."

She won the Amsterdam Marathon in 2002 in her debut at the distance run, but the next year when Wami finally became pregnant, she stopped running immediately, not about to take any risks. Wami started training again a few weeks after Eva was born. Like Radcliffe, she struggled with back injuries. But unlike Radcliffe, it took Wami far longer than nine months to return.

"It was quite difficult," she said. "It was hard to get back into shape."

She ran the New York City Marathon in 2005, thirteen months after Eva was born. She finished seventh in 2:27:40, nearly six minutes slower than her personal best.

Radcliffe had access to pools, extensive equipment, her trusted physical therapist and several doctors when she was preparing for her return from pregnancy. Wami saw a back specialist in Germany, but she mostly saw an Ethiopian doctor and used massage therapy to heal her injuries.

Eventually, she was running stronger than ever. In 2006, she won the Berlin Marathon and in April 2007, she finished second at the London Marathon.

The Berlin Marathon is a flat course. Without the deep pockets of New York and London to recruit a large field, Berlin's officials usually can pay for only one premier athlete each to lead the men's and women's fields. On September 30, 2007, while Gebrselassie made headlines setting his world record of 2:04:26 in Berlin, Wami was certainly no also-ran. She led the women's race from wire to wire, accompanied by the male pacesetter Samuel Woldeammanuel, who was one of her training partners in Ethiopia. Tessema was on a motorcycle beside her for most of the race, shouting occasional encouragement.

Wami was in her own zone, easing up in the final miles to save her legs for New York. She ran 2:23:17 and won $84,000. She had only thirty-five days to recover and train before her next marathon, in New York. Was she ambitious, compulsive or plain crazy to try this feat?

"It's not crazy," Tessema said with a broad grin two hours after she won the Berlin race. "It's courageous."

On the day Wami and her husband returned to Addis Ababa from Berlin, she ran 10 kilometers on a recovery run.

Her training, which she prefers to do alone or with only one or two other runners, takes her 8,000 feet above sea level into forest trails above the capital city. Like any elite marathoner, Wami usually records 140-mile weeks preceding a marathon. But she used

Berlin as a training run and never needed to run that far again before New York.

Between training and parenting, Wami only occasionally has time to bake her own spongy Ethiopian bread known as *injera*; she has help in the kitchen. Like Tulu before her, Wami is changing societal views of women's roles, even if her example is not widely publicized.

In Ethiopia, there are only two daily newspapers, one in English, one in Amharic; they are both only eight pages and both owned by the government. The media culture is starkly different than it is in Great Britain, where the editors fixate on Radcliffe as a personality and an athlete, plastering her on their front and back pages.

The success of Ethiopian women's distance running continues to expand in a country that has celebrated men's distance running since Abebe Bikila ran barefoot to win the marathon gold medal at the 1960 Rome Olympics. Kenenisa Bekele would win his sixth straight cross-country title in March 2008, while Tirunesh Dibaba would win the women's title and her sister, Genzebe, would win the junior women's title. Just three weeks prior to New York, Wami's marathon rival, Berhane Adere, defended her Chicago Marathon title.

"I feel I have inspired other women in what I'm doing," Wami said, "and also, because I have had a child and have gone back to running, I can be an inspiration."

Wami does not race here today to promote her Ethiopian heritage; she runs for her family. That peaceful countenance she has shown since the first mile is an accurate reflection of the contentment she has in her life. If there are children around her, Wami is happy. Like her mother, Wami usually has no fewer than ten people in and out of her house every day—relatives, neighbors and their offspring. Her own daughter, Eva, who is four years old going on 12, with bubbly English-language skills that have surpassed her mother's, is most assuredly the queen of the house. She commands attention but showers affection.

"Gete, she's crazy about kids," Haile Gebrselassie said a few months before the Marathon. Wami is the unofficial aunt to his four children. "When she didn't have kids of her own, she would come to our house to play with my kids," Gebrselassie said, adding with a bemused frown: "She never played with me or my wife."

Gebrselassie is not accustomed to coming in second for any reason. Wami, in his shadow, understands he is king.

B y the Mile 7 marker, Wami is sinking into a trancelike focus just behind Radcliffe. At 10:25 a.m., the Park Slope crowds are not too dense or too loud yet. Toddlers sit on the shoulders of their parents, and fans carrying posters for their loved ones casually fill in the sidewalks, knowing that most of the runners are still at least an hour away. The punk band Fiasco begins to strum a few earnest notes where they have set up at 15th Street. It is all white noise to the professional runners.

Wami looks at Radcliffe's back and uses it as a mark. *Stay with her*, she tells herself. Wami allows herself only one other thought today: Eva. She wonders what her daughter is doing back in Addis Ababa, which is eight hours ahead of New York. Wami wants to win another marathon for her daughter.

The women are about to leave the four-mile straightaway of Fourth Avenue, which has grown increasingly commercial since they crossed 40th Street. They have passed every national fast food chain, rooted like advertisements to reinforce the benefits of exercise and healthy living (but oh, the greasy smell of french fries wafting from the Kentucky Fried Chicken restaurant at 28th Street is so tempting). The Mobil gas station's convenience store at 30th Street seems aptly named just for today: "On the Run." The auto body repair shops are closed. No matter, Wami and Radcliffe's engines are running strong.

They are headed straight for the looming thirty-four-story Williamsburgh Savings Bank, where Fourth Avenue dead-ends at the intersection of Atlantic and Flatbush avenues. For the final two miles of the four-mile stretch on Fourth Avenue, the Bank Building—the tallest structure in Brooklyn—gives runners an easily identifiable landmark on the horizon. Built in 1929, it has had many tenants—from bank offices to dentist offices and now condominiums. Its signature clocks on the tower's four sides have been preserved. Today, they are witnesses to a rivalry in motion.

8

"GONNA FLY NOW"

Mile 8, Lafayette Avenue, Brooklyn

Grunge cover bands without a record label discover an instant audience during the New York City Marathon. Kilted men holding bagpipes stand on a Bay Ridge corner and somehow do not look incongruous on a day when runners are wearing their own costumes. Like switching radio channels, runners quickly hear different, eclectic tunes on the course; each mile of this race fronts an average of five sidewalk bands.

Yet there is something distinctly different about the musical corridor between Mile Markers 8 and 9, certainly something more dynamic and well rehearsed than any of the warm-up acts so far. Appropriately, the tenor of the entertainment changes after passing the Brooklyn Academy of Music, a revered New York landmark since 1861 that has presented a range of artists from progressive to traditional.

Today, the building serves as a silent symbol of harmonic convergence. The orange, blue and green courses that took different ramps off the Verrazano-Narrows Bridge into Brooklyn and ran on different sides of Fourth Avenue now merge at Mile Marker 8, which is just past BAM on Lafayette Avenue.

Here, the sidewalk noise is amplified, and not just by the fans or the thunderous din of plastic noisemakers. Bruce Springsteen's "Born to Run" blasts from speakers (finally a recognizable tune!) and his song serves as a preconcert prelude to what's ahead.

Bishop Loughlin Memorial High School, on Lafayette at Clermont Avenue, is more renowned for its cross-country team and for its band than for being the alma mater of New York City's former mayor Rudolph Giuliani. In the first three of the five-borough marathons, Bishop Loughlin was only a water stop. In 1979, Ed Bowes, the legendary track coach at Loughlin, suggested to the band director, Louis Maffei, that he get his students involved.

So Maffei told the band to prepare for the Marathon and picked the theme to *Rocky*. The song, with its little-used title, "Gonna Fly Now," has become the band's signature, if not the hallmark of sporting inspiration everywhere. Originally consisting of twenty student musicians, the Bishop Loughlin Band now makes Marathon Sunday its homecoming event, drawing 120 students and alumni to play their trumpets, flutes, saxophones, clarinets, keyboards, electric guitars and tubas for more than two continuous hours. The runners shuffle by the band, waving their arms and pumping their fists to the motivational song.

The musicians can't get it out of their head. Maffei acknowledged he had tried to change the repertoire a couple of times, but inevitably gave the running public what it wanted. "It's not something you get sick of," he said a few weeks before the race. "It's an anthem. It's something that doesn't stop."

Nor does Maffei. Today, sweat drips from his black hair, moustache and wire-rimmed glasses as he bounds around in the Marathon shirt he wears over his heavy purple school sweats. "I conduct;

I am out there kicking and screaming—it's a marathon within a marathon," he added.

He and the band members are mesmerized by the athletes in wheelchairs and the costume-clad foreigners; runners smile and often stop to take pictures with the band. "When I look out on the sidewalk," Maffei said, "it's almost like your whole life is in front of you."

To Maffei's life-affirming delight, he will receive thank-you e-mails and letters from marathoners. Henri Greuter, 46, a first-timer from the Netherlands, wrote: "Maybe for all of you, playing the same song over and over again is boring and dull. But you played it at a moment that I could use it very well. Thanks to all of you for being there and performing. That is surely an achievement in itself."

If anyone understands the exhilarating power of "Gonna Fly Now," it is Cindy Peterson. Fifty-five years ago, when she was 13, she really did fly—on Canadian Air Force jump planes. Cindy, who grew up in Montreal, had won a singing contest on the radio program *Call Me Uncle*, a distant forerunner to *American Idol*. She then became a regular on the program before joining the teenage singing troupe, Blue Sky Review. On weekends, the group traveled to military bases, performing all over Canada.

From the time she was nine years old, Cindy was self-conscious about her appearance; singing gave her the confidence to become someone else. "When I got up to sing, I was the ugly duckling turning into the swan," she said. "I would go to school dances where my brother had the band. I'd sing a song and then I'd be asked to dance. It's the inner beauty that comes out."

Cindy turned professional at 16, recording an album and cutting a single, which she sent to the Philadelphia singer Al Alberts, who had founded the Four Aces pop group. Alberts "flipped" over her voice, she said, and he and his wife invited Cindy to stay in their lavish home while she recorded songs. She did a cover of "At Last," an old Glenn Miller tune that was played on *American Bandstand* in the fifties.

Her career was thriving and Cindy at 19 years old did not think about widening her social circle. But one day a cousin suggested that Cindy meet a neighbor who was a handsome car salesman in New Jersey. Six months later Cindy and William Robert Peterson were married. When Cindy was selected for a U.S.O. tour with Bob Hope that would go to Hawaii, her husband was upset. He turned to her and said: "Make a choice. Either be with me, or go travel and sing."

She stayed with him for thirteen years.

"It was the worst thing I did in my life," she said. "When I got married, I didn't think he was going to stop my career. It was like taking my right arm away."

After their divorce Cindy, then 32, resumed her singing career, working with local big bands and performing at weddings. By then, she was living in central New Jersey and had a full-time job working at the Chicago Title Insurance company to support her two sons. She was tagged to become a saleswoman but had no experience, so she ordered motivational tapes. The tapes suggested she write a "life list" of thirty goals.

She put the list in a suitcase, which she forgot about until 1992. When she discovered the list, Cindy realized she had fulfilled all but two goals. She crossed off "Buy a Jaguar" since she drove a company car. But she circled the final goal: run a marathon.

At the time, she was 20 pounds overweight and had never run before. Inspired by the widely publicized story of Fred Lebow running the 1992 Marathon while in remission from cancer, Cindy told herself: "Time to get moving."

She ran the 1994 New York City Marathon in 5:42:31. The following year, she was one of five women who formed a running club for women 50 years and older, the Mercury Masters.

Cindy became addicted to the marathon, and its ability to open new worlds for her. Over the last fourteen years, she has run thirty-five marathons on five continents. In 1996, she recorded her personal best in her hometown marathon in Montreal, where she ran 4:45, with a sling over a wrist she had broken. She ran the Antarctica Marathon on a cruise ship in 2001, the year the race was canceled on land due to inclement weather. Instead, it was held on the ship's decks, and she completed it on the cramped middle deck despite banging into other runners and lifeboats.

Cindy ran in China, where a course marshal tried to tear off her number because he told her the course was closed after three hours instead of five. She dodged the marshal and, together with three friends, finished in five hours anyway.

She took her grandson, Matthew, 12, to Rome, and he ran the last four miles with her when she was limping and bleeding after tripping over a discarded garbage bag at the start of the race. Seeing her injured, he arranged for a stretcher at the finish line.

Matthew not only accompanied her on other marathon trips to France and Norway, but he became her personal assistant when she started a DJ business, Singing Cindy DJs. Cindy became known in central New Jersey as the Glamorous Grandma, or Glam Gram.

For Marathon Sunday, she has sewn the letters of her name onto a rectangle of wicking material that she recycles for every marathon. On her head is her trademark sequined purple and red hat, perfectly matching her purple and red Mercury Masters shirt. She is in costume, performing again.

Her twin passions of music and marathons conjoin as she runs through the streets of New York, enabling her to replicate her sense of fulfillment. "I have accomplished in running what I was accomplishing in singing," she said.

Today, Cindy has a new race strategy. She is recovering from rotator cuff surgery in July and could not train intensively. She decides, along with her friends in the Mercury Masters, to run one mile and then walk for a mile, doing a variation of running guru Jeff Galloway's injury-free plan. Eight miles into the race, the plan is working perfectly.

Cindy feels inspired not only by the company of her teammates, but by the music and fans along the course. She feels as if she is onstage again. "You need that applause, you need that audience," she said, "and running gives you that."

For years, Emmanuel Baptist Church, five blocks down the road from Bishop Loughlin, had trouble drawing people to services on Marathon Sunday. The noise outside distracted the worshippers. Finally, the congregation's leaders decided if they could not fight the Marathon, they would join in.

This year, groups of twelve singers at a time from the 120-member choir come outside to harmonize on the church's steps. Dressed in black robes with brilliant scarves of African kente cloth, they sing twenty-one songs, all upbeat urban spirituals that appeal to the runners.

"As far as we see it, the whole Christian life is a marathon," said Frank Haye, the pastor of music and arts at Emmanuel Baptist.

He explained that this is evidenced in a modern interpretation of the passage from Ecclesiastes 9:11: "The race is not won by the swift nor the strong, but to he who endures in the end."

Said Haye: "Life is a process, with ups and downs, trials and tribulations, and you cannot give up.

"That's what the runners are doing out there, from the professional runners to those who just want to try it before they die. We want to encourage anybody to finish the race, because that is your reward."

The Reverend Timothy Wright, the founder of Brooklyn's Grace Tabernacle Christian Center, wrote the lyrics to one spiritual hymn, "We're Gonna Make It," nearly two decades ago. The message is just as relevant today: "I know somehow, and I know some way, we're going to make it. No matter the test, whatever comes our way, we're going to make it."

As they hear the joyful gospel harmonies, runners raise their hands and clap, participating in the interactive rituals of the African-American church. "We felt we were going out to bless the people running," Haye will say later. "But what started happening was we were blessed."

9

THE KENYAN MYSTIQUE

Mile 9, Entering Bed-Stuy, Brooklyn

Hendrick Ramaala has just led the pack on a wild goose chase through Brooklyn, sprinting Miles 7 and 8 at a combined pace of 9:11—a foot speed of 13 miles an hour. His surge does nothing to shake off any of the dozen elite runners, eight of whom are from Kenya, including the 29-year-old favorite, Martin Lel.

As Lel passes the brownstones, redbrick apartments, housing project towers and four-story tenements of the Bedford-Stuyvesant neighborhood—the largest African-American community in New York City—he sees small groups of people congregating on their stoops and standing casually on the sidewalk. This is more humanity than Lel encounters in a 10-mile radius when he is at home.

Lel lives in the temperate and lush Rift Valley of Kenya, in a secluded area in western Kenya that is a loosely incorporated village named Kimngeru. It is just 15 miles from the major city of Eldoret (with a population of about 200,000). Go north from Eldoret's outskirts, turn off the main paved road and wind down a dirt road into wooded hills to get to Lel's two-story, six-room house. It is made of both mud and stone, with a blue iron-sheeted roof and a satellite dish. His brothers live there when he is out of town competing. His house sits near a loose cluster of three stores that resemble shacks, one church, one school and a scattering of other houses spread through the wooded hills.

Lel belongs to the Nandi subgroup of the Kalenjin tribe, to which more than three-quarters of Kenya's elite runners belong. By the time he was 10 years old, Lel knew he wanted to be a runner and follow in his tribe's tradition. Running is the ticket out of hunger and poverty in Kenya; it is a birthright for the Kalenjin.

Lel believes that more than anything about growing up in the Rift Valley—the starchy diet or the altitude of 5,000 to 10,000 feet above sea level or the long runs to school—the Kalenjin warrior heritage is what makes Kenyan runners so successful. For nearly 1,000 years in the Rift Valley, the Kalenjin were known for their military organization and their cattle herding culture. They fiercely protected their land from other tribes, a practice that would continue through British colonial rule in the 1950s, and sadly, through the political violence between the Kalenjin and Kikuyu tribes that erupted after the flawed presidential elections of December 2007.

Lel, however, chooses to focus on the centuries-old traditions of his ancestors. "The Kalenjin warriors would run 100 kilometers at a time, sometimes surviving without food for 50 or 60 kilometers," he said. "This character is in the people; it is in our genetic type. We are very resistant and have such a strong system. We have that extra energy in our bodies."

Kipchoge Keino, a Kalenjin, won the gold medal in the 1,500 meters at the 1968 Mexico City Olympic Games, despite running with a severely infected gall bladder. His victory would spawn a running generation in his tribe and an unspoken philosophy: running with pain must not only be accepted, it is the only way to glory.

Lel's path began like that of so many other Kenyan champions:

on the road to school. Lel ran nearly 24 miles every day to and from his primary school—just two kilometers shy of a marathon. Lel said he did not notice the distance or the 200-kilometer weeks he logged from the time he was nine years old.

"Many people come from the same village. We all were together, talking; it was not a big deal," he said.

Yet at the time, Lel thought those twice-a-day workouts were not enough for him. He spent his lunch hour training on his own. A teacher spotted him and reprimanded him, but in a constructive way; the teacher told Lel that in order to strengthen his body to be a runner he had to eat at mealtime.

When he finished school, Lel did not pursue a full-time running career, nor did he follow his father's career as an itinerant preacher. Instead, Lel trained while working at a small grocery store near his house. He saved enough money to open his own store down the road. Calling it a store rather overstates Lel's business, which he still operates (at no profit) despite his international marathon success. The store is more like a stand, with a roof and walls that seem ready to contradict even that word. He sells staples like flour, sugar and Coca-Cola out of the window of a shack not big enough for people to enter.

Lel's business mission was not to become rich but to help his neighbors. His career changed in 2002, though, when he entered a half-marathon in Eldoret at age 23. "I didn't win," Lel recalled. He finished in 1 hour, 3 minutes, which was only good enough for fifteenth place in a field of six hundred runners. "I really knew I could do something better," he said.

A cousin put him in contact with an Italian agent, Federico Rosa, who represented many Kenyan runners. Lel concentrated on training rather than his business, and within a year he was excelling on the half-marathon circuit. The marathon was his next territory to conquer, and Lel's biggest breakthrough came in 2003 when he won the New York City Marathon (in 2:10:30). He returned to Kenya and built a house for his parents. He gave cows to neighbors in need, supplied them with sugar and flour. Because he saw himself as a man of the people, he refused to buy a fancy car, instead keeping a modest one with a driver only to negotiate Kenya's hazardous dirt roads.

Since Lel's first success in New York, people in Eldoret have frequently come to him for assistance, which has proved to be both a blessing and a burden. The poverty depresses him. "In Africa," he said, "sometimes I feel like crying."

Lel knows that in order to help relatives and friends, he must continue to win. But earlier in his career he had trouble sustaining his success on road and track from the spring and summer seasons; many times he found himself injured by the time he got to his fall marathon of choice—New York. He pulled out of the 2006 race a month before with a torn hamstring, the same injury that stopped him from competing in 2004. In 2005, he flew to New York but was struggling with a strained muscle in his lower right leg and pulled out the night before the race.

He sat in the bleachers at the finish line, instead, watching Ramaala and fellow Kenyan Paul Tergat storm together uphill in the final 385 yards in Central Park. And then he saw Tergat win after he leaned past a tumbling Ramaala at the tape. Tergat came over to hug Lel, and more than just sweat rubbed off. Tergat had taught his younger countryman an important lesson, and Lel made a mental note: *I can win with my kick.*

"That was a day," Lel recalled, "where I got my experience."

The Kenyan runners created their mystique by dominating big-city marathons, and rival runners have only perpetuated it.

Kenyans train together in their homeland in packs, sharing the lead to pace one another during long runs the way they work together in a race. That can be daunting for a runner who is the only representative of his country.

"People lose confidence just because they are Kenyan," Ramaala said. "On the starting line, very fit guys are looking like they are losing it."

This sense of intimidation does not track with Ramaala's life philosophy: *You have to believe you can win—or else why run?*

"They have two legs just like the rest of us," Ramaala likes to say.

Their legs just happen to have had more success in the marathon than those of any other nation. According to the International Association of Athletics Federations (IAAF), in 2007, male runners from Kenya produced 429 marathon finishes of 2:18 or faster. The same year, a total of twenty-four running times of 2:18 or faster belonged to U.S. runners, fifteen were produced by South African marathoners. Kenya is a country roughly the size of Texas; South Africa is twice Kenya's size.

The domination in New York is obvious. Coming into today's race, Kenyan men have won six of the last ten years; Kenyan women have won five of the last thirteen years here.

Kenyan runners did not just arrive at the finish line overnight. Originally they came to the United States in the seventies and eighties on college athletic scholarships. Joseph Nzau, an All-American at the University of Wyoming from 1977 to 1982, was the first Kenyan to win a major international marathon, the 1983 Chicago Marathon. Ibrahim Hussein, who ran for the University of New Mexico, won the New York Marathon in 1987 (he now serves as secretary of Kenya's athletics federation). Kenya's Douglas Wakiihuri won New York in 1990, but he had lived and trained in Japan.

That year, 1990, Kenya's running scene changed dramatically.

Mike Boit, a former top 800-meter runner and later the country's sports commissioner, helped change the rules that had restricted athletes' travel outside of Africa. He opened the doors both ways, allowing runners to compete internationally and foreign agents to come to Kenya to work with athletes.

The first wave of Kenyan-trained winners in New York started with the tiny, mighty Tegla Loroupe, who won the women's race in 1994 and 1995. At 4 foot 11 and weighing only 85 pounds, Loroupe provided Kenyans with an example of a woman who refused to adhere to traditional gender roles that held them in a position of inferiority.

Two years later, Kenya's John Kagwe ignited the men's wave in New York by winning back-to-back Marathon titles in 1997 and 1998. Every year since, at least one Kenyan has finished among the top three in New York.

Ramaala said he can understand Kenyan runners, because he trained with them early in his career. In the late fall of 1996, his British agent, John Bicourt, arranged for the 24-year-old Ramaala to travel to London and work with his Kenyan athletes. Ramaala observed their camaraderie in training and cooking. He ate *ugali*, the traditional starchy Kenyan staple that tastes like porridge and is rich in carbohydrates but not in fat. It is similar to the porridge of corn meal Ramaala grew up eating in his village in South Africa.

Ramaala discovered that he and the Kenyans shared a similar metaphorical hunger, born out of a real-life one. In 1983, Ramaala and everyone in his South African village endured a famine. They had to eat maize that was dropped from airplanes by relief organizations. The grain packets were supposed to be free; but certain people in the village quickly snatched them away and made them available only on the black market. Ramaala shuddered when recalling how he had to eat maize, a poor substitute for corn meal or flour that tasted to him like cement. Ramaala was a teenager, helping to care for his younger siblings, and he had to ration the family's food.

A decade later, when he went to live and train with Kenyan runners, Ramaala was still relatively new to the sport. He was dazzled by the simple orchestration of their group runs, how they worked together and then how they completed their task without complaint—be it a tempo run or hill repeats. "They just go out and execute," he said.

But for someone as perceptive as Ramaala, the experience helped him scout his opponent. "I know their weak points, their strong points," he said.

The Kenyan runners have weak points?

Ramaala hesitated. He said sometimes the pack slows its pace and provides an opening. Then he can shoot through the opening to place himself in position to win. Like the 2005 race in New York when he almost beat Tergat.

"I know that Paul has the better C.V., the faster times. He's a 2:04 and I'm a 2:06," Ramaala said of their respective marathon personal bests (in 2006, his would be 2:06:55 at London).

"One of these days," Ramaala remembered telling himself before the 2005 race, "I'm going to take Paul out."

He paused before adding with his wry smile: "I was going to feel that good about it."

Instead, Ramaala bruised his body and his pride by stumbling to the ground at the finish that year, losing by three-hundredths of a second, which is still the closest men's finish in New York City Marathon history. It produced a memorable photo, which appeared on souvenir posters, postcards and in magazines. That postcard sits on the second shelf of Ramaala's kitchen in Johannesburg, behind mugs and old mail.

Each time he comes to New York, Ramaala must answer questions about 2005. Three days before this race, Ramaala patiently complimented Tergat and said that at least he was beaten by a friend. But after one more question, Ramaala finally shrugged, smiled wearily and said: "Let the past be the past."

At 35, Ramaala knows he may not have many marathons left.

"I was hoping to win some more," Ramaala said almost wistfully. For that reason, he runs this race—if not every race—with a carpe diem attitude.

"If you are ready, you have to grab that opportunity. Don't wait. Because the next year may not be your time. When it's the marathon, I have to try everything to be first. Because it might be my last."

"I know when to take the initiative," he added. "When I'm there, my mind can take it."

Tim Noakes admires Ramaala's mind-set. Noakes, a professor of exercise and sports science at the University of Cape Town, is currently studying the importance of training the brain to produce better performances. Noakes used Ramaala as an example during his inspirational speech to the South African rugby team before the Springboks left for the 2007 Rugby World Cup.

New Zealand was considered the favorite. Noakes implored South Africa's rugby team not to think of the odds but to consider Ramaala's philosophy of running against the more-favored Kenyans.

"I told them what he says: 'If you don't believe you're going to win the race, then you shouldn't be in it.' You have to believe in yourself before the first match begins," Noakes said.

In September and October, while preparing to go to New York,

Ramaala watched every match of his beloved Springboks during the World Cup—all the way to their championship victory.

At Mile Marker 9 in today's race, Ramaala and Lel are part of a pack of runners more than a dozen strong, and they have settled into a comfortable 5:03 pace, appearing to float above the street. At 5 foot 7 and a lean 122 pounds (typical for a runner), Lel possesses a powerful grace in his stride. He barely expresses emotion on the course—unless Ramaala draws it out of him in bursts of speed or conversation.

The next four miles of the Marathon course will feature some sharp turns and narrow streets, so sprinting will not be an option. Besides, an elite runner knows little can be accomplished in these early miles. Brooklyn is a testing ground. Queens is a way station. And Manhattan is where the race gets interesting.

For now, with three miles left in Brooklyn, the elites are jockeying for position, saving their energy for the remaining two-thirds of the race. They have the streets to themselves, unaware of the avalanche behind them.

Amateur marathoners rush toward an important, but unmarked milestone in this stretch: to complete one-third of the race. The topography so far has not been too taxing with its wide avenues and gentle hills. The crowded course is the most challenging part of the race now, and runners have been jostling each other for position over the last 9 miles. The density of the field has not thinned much since runners waited up to fifty minutes to cross the starting line on the lower deck of the Verrazano-Narrows Bridge. That was Marci Glotzer's experience. She is doing her best to keep her 9:30

pace while not slamming into other runners, many of whom do not speak English and others still who are oblivious because they are running with headphones.

To ensure the safety of runners, USA Track & Field, the national governing body of the sport, established a rule in 2006 that prohibits wearing headphones during races. Still, New York Road Runners officials knew they would not be able to enforce the rule, nor did they even try, since the volume of runners is simply too overwhelming.

But headphone wearers are not the troublemakers today. Like multitasking drivers, runners talking on cell phones pose far more of a safety hazard.

Glotzer, a 41-year-old New Yorker running for Fred's Team, later reported on her blog:

"There were so many people on the phone DURING THE MARATHON that I almost started yelling at them, but I didn't want to waste the energy. Now, I don't mean those who call ahead to the people waiting for them to alert them, 'I'm three blocks away!' That's cool."

No, what upsets Glotzer most is the actual conversation she cannot help but overhear from a woman runner who acts like she is out on a Sunday errand, shouting and breathing hard into the phone:

"Hello? Oh hi! How are you? What's up? Good. Oh really? Wow. No, I'm running the marathon now. Marathon. The marathon—26 miles. Yeah, I'm running it right now. So, what's new?"

The woman on the phone starts weaving all over the place, paying no attention to other runners, like Marci, trying to move past her.

Marci shakes her head in annoyance, later scolding the woman in her blog: "And it's 26 POINT TWO, you moron."

Apparently not everybody can appreciate the sanctity of the experience. Or perhaps this cell phone–wielding woman was just trying to place her focus elsewhere, rather than on the fact that two-thirds of the race still remained. It is in Brooklyn's middle miles today where runners are almost relaxed, after the heart-pounding exhilaration of the start has worn off and before the muscle stiffness and blisters begin to set in. The noonday sun still beams overhead, even as clouds begin to encroach on the horizon.

10

A MODEST MILE

Mile 10, Bedford Avenue, Williamsburg

I f the Marathon is a religion, then Fred Lebow was the New York City Marathon's chief rabbi. To some—including his own Orthodox Jewish family—his missionary zeal to promote the race might have seemed sacrilegious, but to Lebow, directing the Marathon gave his life meaning and purpose. In turn, he wanted everyone to experience this joy—even if they could not run.

How, then, to convince the masses to embrace the sport of distance running, one that had no natural arena? The motto Lebow formulated in the late seventies became the model for major city marathons around the world: "Don't bring the people to the race," Lebow said. "Bring the race to the people."

It worked. Nearly everywhere, that is, except the one place that mattered deeply to Lebow. What happens when the people do not really want the race?

The question speaks to the conflict between tradition and innovation, an argument played out not only along the course in the Hasidic Jewish neighborhood of Brooklyn's Bedford Avenue, but also within Lebow himself.

When the runners reach Mile 10 today, they are met with silence, interrupted only by the rustling of the fall leaves on the street or the muted sounds of small hands clapping. The runners see stares—quizzical, blank or bored—or they see people look away in modesty. This portion of Williamsburg, Brooklyn, was the one area where Fred Lebow, born Fishl Lebowitz into an Orthodox Jewish family in Arad, Romania, could not convert the people.

He tried.

During the early eighties, Lebow would shout *"Vasser, vasser!"* from his pace car, telling the people (with his Romanian inflection) in Yiddish to bring water to the runners. At the time, he was overjoyed when they complied. He shouted to them, still in Yiddish, to cheer on the runners. He did elicit spirit from the bemused spectators at times. He even had the No Parking signs printed in Yiddish, to tell residents to remove their cars for the race.

Lebow's passion for such a secular cause, however, never fully took hold in the religious community. And after his death in 1994 of brain cancer, there was no one to promote a personal connection—let alone shout in Yiddish.

"We're in no way going to tell anybody not to run," said Rabbi David Niederman a few weeks before the Marathon. He is the director of the United Jewish Organizations, based in Williamsburg. "If you're asking me, do we feel it's the appropriate place to do that? Within a very strict conservative community, the answer is no. I hope they can find another place to do that.

"There's a reason why there was no running in Williamsburg before it was the promised land for the rest of the world. We wanted to continue our insular shtetl life that we have," he said.

It is as if the runners today, having passed through nearly nine miles of exuberant fans, blaring music and colorful signs, travel on Bedford Avenue into the nineteenth century. The community of the ultra-Orthodox Satmar sect lives along Bedford Avenue. Children peek out of the windows of overcrowded apartments or stand on the stoops to see the Marathon traipse by their block. Men wear black hats, long beards with hanging sidelocks (*peius*) and tzitzit (prayer shawl fringes that serve as symbolic reminders of faith) from their belt loops. The women have children at their long skirts. Children do not cheer or hold signs, though a few young boys and girls offer cups of water. Mostly, people go about their business, talking on cell phones, or crossing the street while occasionally glancing as the spectacle passes.

Sunday is a weekday for the Hasidic community, a day when people work and children attend school. Street closures disrupt bus schedules, and cars are still towed the night before, despite those signs in Yiddish.

"Not that we're against it—what could be wrong with it?" said a deli owner along Bedford Avenue, who always loses business on Marathon Sunday. "It's just not our style."

Beyond the inconvenience factor, the Marathon runs counter to the Hasidic community's strict interpretation of the commandment of *tzniut*, modesty. "We are not going to encourage people to look at immodesty in our sense," Rabbi Niederman explained.

Men and women run the race side by side, and such intermingling is prohibited in public places by the ultra-Orthodox community. Women are not supposed to look at scantily clad men, while men should not look at women whose outfits leave legs, arms and stomachs bare.

"They have their main interest in establishing themselves as heroes in this field. It is not exactly what the Hasidic Jews are all about," said Rabbi Joseph Weber, of Yeshiva Kehilath Yaakov in Williamsburg.

Weber explained that paying attention to running or engaging in strenuous exercise is a distraction from studying the Torah. Still, two seminal Jewish scholars, Rabbi Akiba in the second century and Moses Maimonides, the twelfth-century philosopher, advocated taking care of one's body.

In the Satmar world of Bedford Avenue, the Marathon is not a matter of Talmudic debate, but instead a matter of private discussion, if at all. One mother could only marvel at what Paula Radcliffe has been able to accomplish: have a baby and within nine months return to her career as a runner.

"I wish I could run the marathon—it has always been my dream," said a Hasidic woman, very pregnant, in her late twenties, as she shopped at a local grocery store. "But that is not something we do."

Softly, she explained that she would have to run while wearing her wig and skirt, with her arms and legs fully covered. Sometimes, when she and her husband take a couple of days away together, she enjoys a run along a boardwalk. For now, she said with a smile, there are children to look after, a life to lead. She still loves watching the race, as she did as a child living along Bedford Avenue. She used to hand out water to the runners. "We're all very proud of them," she said.

Despite attempting to separate themselves from the profane world around them though, the Hasidim on Bedford Avenue might unintentionally and quite subtly be establishing a bond with the very people who run through their shtetl. Their strict adherence to the laws of Torah and self-discipline share a sense of extremism that a disciplined runner knows all too well.

At first, Lebow's own Orthodox family did not understand his fervor for the sport. Lebow kept kosher and attended some holidays with his family, but otherwise was not an observant Jew. His family was disappointed that he had distanced himself from his strict Orthodox heritage.

As the second-youngest child of seven, Lebow survived the Holocaust as a teenager by hiding in Bulgaria and Romania. But because the Russians occupied his hometown of Arad, Romania, after the war, his parents sent him and his older brother, Mike, to the former Czechoslovakia. From there, the brothers went to England and on to Ireland, where they stayed and studied in Orthodox schools. Lebow wrote in his autobiography, *Inside the World of Big-Time Marathoning*, that in order to earn money as a teenage refugee, he became a diamond smuggler. Allan Steinfeld, Lebow's close friend and successor to the presidency of the New York Road Runners club, said he heard Lebow tell this story more than once. But Lebow's siblings, concerned about Lebow's legacy, said he made up that story just to make the publisher happy.

The spirit of the story was true to his personality, however.

"From an early age," Lebow wrote, "I was learning about living by your wits, always being on your toes, improvising."

When he was 19, Lebow left Ireland with Mike for a Talmudic academy in Brooklyn, but the school felt as oppressive to Lebow as his yeshiva in Eastern Europe. After Lebow spent a year at another religious school in Kansas City, he went to live with Mike in Cleveland. There, he changed his name from Lebowitz to Lebow and became part owner of an improvisational comedy club called the Left-Handed Compliment.

In 1962, Lebow moved to New York, where he worked in the garment industry making knockoffs. He began running in 1966 after he had struggled to play tennis and his roommate, Brian Crawford, challenged him to a race around the Central Park reservoir. Lebow ran his first official race in 1969, a five-miler that was eleven laps around Yankee Stadium in the Bronx, and was instantly hooked. He started attending events put on by the Road Runners club, and the following year he ran his first marathon, also in the Bronx.

By that point, Lebow had taken a leadership role in the club and convinced the other members—namely the president, Vince Chiappetta—that it was time to hold a marathon in Central Park. He and Chiappetta codirected the original New York City Marathon, which took place on September 13, 1970. In 1972, Lebow became president of the New York Road Runners club, a job he performed vigorously until his death in 1994.

With the conviction of a long-distance runner and an outsider's appreciation of a group that would welcome anyone with a pair of sneakers, Lebow made the New York City Marathon his life. He was an immigrant with a heavy accent, but through his Marathon, Lebow found a fast track to assimilation.

"He was married to the Marathon, which upset my parents very much," said his sister, Sarah Katz, who lives north of New York City in the ultra-Orthodox community of Monsey, New York.

When Lebow gushed about the Marathon to his parents, who also immigrated to Brooklyn, he told them that it was not just the race or the event itself that was so important. "It is the people around the Marathon," Lebow always said.

One day his sister asked him, "Why do you care so much about strangers?"

Lebow responded by invoking one of Judaism's most basic tenets: "There is no such thing as a stranger; every human being is special."

Sarah remembered how one day a woman came running up to Lebow on the street. "I can't thank you enough," the woman told Lebow. "My mother suffered from depression. She started to run and now she's doing fantastic."

The rest of the day Lebow was on a high.

"His whole thing was to make people happy," Sarah added. "He got people volunteering for nothing, for maybe a T-shirt."

People seemed to flock to Lebow, whether he was traveling overseas or around New York. His thick beard identified him just as much as the painter's cap and track suit he always wore.

"I saw Fred as the pied piper of running," Steinfeld said. "He was evangelical about the Marathon. He saw it as the great equalizer, that anybody could do it."

As enthusiastic as Lebow was about his race, he was just as possessive about it. He ran board meetings with a heavy hand and took offense when anyone tried to disrupt the race. Lebow may not have always been diplomatic, but he was extremely clever.

For the second five-borough race in 1977, Lebow changed the Marathon course to go away from the Brooklyn Navy Yard because the area was too remote; he decided to bring the race instead through the wider and more populated thoroughfare of Bedford Avenue. However that plan did not please gang leaders from the Bedford-Stuyvesant neighborhood, which borders the religious blocks of Bedford, because they thought the race would infringe on their turf. The leaders confronted Lebow in his office and immediately he turned the situation to his advantage. He bribed the gang with New York City Marathon T-shirts, jackets and hats, in exchange for them policing their corner of the course. He made them feel important, and they never disturbed the race.

Lebow took a more solemn approach with the leaders of the Satmar Hasidic community when he first changed the course such that it would infringe on their neighborhood. He spoke to them in Yiddish, told them who his family was back in Arad. Lebow's older brother Schlomo was a rabbi in another section of Williamsburg. Once the community leaders recognized his connections, they gave him their tacit support.

Lebow had wanted to bring the runners to the people—notably to *his* people, who contributed to the ethnic diversity of the city. "Fred was a New Yorker from Romania," said George Hirsch, the chairman of the board of New York Road Runners. "He understood New York was this kind of a magnet."

Like a true New Yorker, Lebow had chutzpah. He was charming at times, bluntly honest at others. He cared little for material things, or at least buying them. He bragged how he never had to buy shoes or track suits, since sponsors provided them. He rented an apartment on East 53rd Street for sixty-nine dollars a month.

Lebow was as demanding as a boss, sometimes driven by the impossible, sometimes impossibly driven. He drew hard bargaining lines when negotiating with elite runners like Bill Rodgers and Alberto Salazar and former New York mayor Edward Koch.

In the late seventies and early eighties, Lebow battled with Koch on two fronts: admitting athletes in wheelchairs and paying the top runners appearance fees to lure them to New York. Since the sport was still considered amateur, Lebow was paying athletes under the table but not hiding it. This incensed Koch, because he thought it was hypocritical and potentially bad for the city's image.

"I probably was wrong, but that was my feeling and I expressed it to him," Koch recalled in his office a few weeks before the Marathon. "But he didn't listen anyway. He was paying those bounties after I had said that we would not do it."

Koch admitted in retrospect maybe Lebow had a point. "He kept the race the number-one race, because undoubtedly Boston or the others would have taken that title away from us."

Koch added: "Having lived through the Holocaust, he was someone who had enormous intestinal strength. It was no issue that he would ever accept a defeat on. He had enormous heart and strength and intellect."

Lebow thrived on showmanship and shtick, and one of his early promotional efforts helped forge the legend of both Alberto Salazar and the New York Marathon. When Lebow first recruited Salazar to run the Marathon as a college track star, he thrust an entry form in Salazar's hands during the 1980 Olympic Trials in Eugene, Oregon. The form asked Salazar to predict his running time in New York. Salazar wrote that he would run sub–2:10. Lebow turned the answer into headlines, and Salazar, for his part, did not back off his claim. In 1980 he won in 2:09:42—the fastest debut marathon for an American. The following year, Salazar set a world record in New York. He would win for a third consecutive year in 1982.

"The thing about Fred was, he wasn't just the New York City Marathon race director," Salazar said. "He was an ambassador who loved running."

During track and field meets—even though Lebow was not organizing them—Salazar remembered how Lebow would often position himself in the infield, and yell and scream like crazy over an exciting race. He would attend other races to bring back ideas for his own. Lebow was never satisfied, always searching for innovations to improve the runners' experience and ways to court new sponsors.

Despite attracting hundreds of thousands of runners to the sport, Lebow, though, felt he failed much closer to home. He was sad he could not convince his brothers or sister to partake in what he created. It was not until the year he died that he learned his nephew had decided to honor him by training for the Marathon. Moshe Katz, Sarah's son, ran the November 1994 race, in what was the Marathon's twenty-fifth anniversary. Lebow died on October 9.

Today, most runners only know Lebow from his bronze statue at the East 90th Street entrance to Central Park, a block away from the offices of the New York Road Runners. They may not know that there were bureaucratic snarls with the city and Central Park just to get the statue erected, and that there were also religious objections from Lebow's own family who held firm to the strict Orthodox law against graven images. The night before the statue was unveiled, November 4, 1994, a rabbi had to chisel a chip between the statue's left forefinger and thumb, thus making the likeness an imperfect representation of God's creation.

The enduring image of Lebow is not in bronze, however, but in marathon lore surrounding his 1992 run. Lebow had participated in 69 marathons around the world, including the 1970 race in Central Park, but until then he had never participated in the five-borough race. Determined to fulfill a promise he made to himself, Lebow started training once his cancer was in remission, following two years of chemotherapy. His doctors advised him only to participate and not necessarily finish, but that kind of thinking was against Lebow's brand of marathon religion.

He chose for his running partner that day the nine-time New York champion Grete Waitz, who had become a close friend over the years. During the race, she made Lebow walk every couple of miles. While the pace was painful for her—she was used to running the course in just under 2 hours and 30 minutes—Waitz would say it was her most memorable New York City Marathon. She and Lebow finished together in 5 hours, 32 minutes and 34 seconds, holding their hands up high, crying and then falling into a hug. Lebow kissed the ground at the finish line; he had already felt the embrace from New Yorkers throughout the day as they applauded his courage.

"Running was just so important to him," Steinfeld said. "When he went out there to train, he just ran his ass off. That's what he wanted to do; he wanted to feel alive."

When Waitz, a school teacher from Oslo, ran her first marathon in New York back in 1978, she remembered little about the city—except Williamsburg. "That got my attention," she recalled. "I had never seen Orthodox Jews before, and I thought they had dressed up in costumes."

When she told Lebow this after the race—which she won, setting a world record in the process—he just laughed kindly and explained the Hasidic community's rules for strict living.

Thirty years later, runners still find the neighborhood intriguing for its stark difference from the rest of the course. Harrie Bakst, his brother, Rich, and their family belong to an Orthodox synagogue in Riverdale, New York, but they are not observant. They cannot read the Hebrew on some store signs or the Yiddish parking directions. Today, Harrie sees one Hasidic girl holding out water, but since he has just taken a cup at an official stop, he simply smiles, shakes his head and continues on his journey.

11

"AIN'T NO STOPPING US NOW"

Mile 11, Williamsburg

Tattoo artists near Mile Marker 11 signal a sea change on Bedford Avenue as runners head north into twenty-first-century Williamsburg, home to hipsters, art galleries, coffee houses, antique clothing stores, and fancy pizza places. What was once German is now gentrified: That's Brooklyn.

Along the street, the Metropolitan Pool still stands as an oasis to an earlier age. Designed in 1922 by the architect Henry Bacon, the pristinely restored neoclassic building, clad in brick with a vaulted skylight, draws neighbors to its lap lanes. On this morning, the pool's staff and volunteers have set up speakers on the outside steps, prepared water and blown up balloons. "Chariots of Fire" plays from the speakers, unintentionally saluting the UK's Paula Radcliffe. That film was about a 100-meter race in England; its theme song is now synonymous with slow-motion parodies.

Radcliffe and Gete Wami race by at 11 miles an hour. Sweat forms on their foreheads, but their ponytails are still perfectly taut, neither showing signs of breaking any time soon. Their speed is still slower than that of the elite athletes who passed by an hour earlier, athletes who give off an entirely different kinetic energy.

The elite men racing custom-made wheelchairs average speeds of 18 miles an hour—topping out at 35 miles an hour downhill—while the elite wheelchair women average 15 to 16 miles an hour during the race. With their legs tucked into their sleek, three-wheel racing chairs, and their heads hidden inside colorful helmets, they seem to be floating in their own sphere.

That bubble bursts when the wheelers hit potholes, clip crevices on the bridges or career around 180-degree turns coming off those bridges—with only a shallow bank of hay bales to brace them if they should hurtle off course. These obstacles make New York arguably the hardest wheelchair marathon in the world. For now, on this slightly downhill straightaway in Brooklyn between Miles 11 and 12, the racers are settling into a comfortable rhythm.

Dorothy Exum, an employee of the Metropolitan Pool and a New Yorker for fifty years, witnesses her first Marathon live. She stands in amazement when the wheelers pass by. "They're awesome. I applaud them most of all," Exum will say.

It is as if Exum's favorite song that today, the popular soul-disco tune from McFadden and Whitehead, gives voice especially to the men and women racing: *Ain't no stopping us now, we're on the move/ Ain't no stopping us now, we got the groove.*

The wheelchair athletes' disabilities—whether by accident, by birth or by childhood affliction—become afterthoughts to them. Winning takes priority. Powering their chairs solely with their arms and hands, these athletes compete around the world as often as two, even three races a month just to earn a living. Besides the five marathon majors, Atlanta's Peachtree 10K, the Honolulu Marathon and the Oita, Japan, Marathon have become popular on the wheelchair racing circuit.

Prize money, however, is but a fraction of what the able-bodied competitors earn. The first-place prize for a runner in New York is $140,000. The first-place prize for a push-rim wheeler is $7,500 (thanks to sponsorship from Avis), plus an additional $5,000 for a course record.

All of the top racers in the sport are in New York today—there are thirty-two of them in the men's division but just ten in the women's division. "It's hard to get together a large group who do marathons, and it's even more difficult to get an elite group of women together," said Amanda McGrory, the 2006 New York champion, who at 21 is still a student at the University of Illinois.

She also competes on a wheelchair basketball team, but because there are no NCAA (National Collegiate Athletic Association) restrictions for wheelchair athletes, McGrory can collect prize money from wheelchair racing. As a collegian, she might be the only elite wheeler who thinks of the prize money as a windfall. "I use it to get to my next competition," she said.

At 35, Edith Hunkeler is the superstar of the sport but still works a second job, as an administrator for a jeweler back in her native Switzerland. An effervescent blonde who bears more than a little resemblance to model Christie Brinkley, Hunkeler is a two-time New York and Boston Marathon champion.

Two accidents, twelve years apart, have only made her more determined.

Growing up on a farm in Altishofen, a village of 2,000 people near Lucerne, Hunkeler always played sports with her two younger brothers, swimming, bicycling, skiing and walking everywhere.

In 1994, she was driving to work alone one morning when she was struck from behind by a car at a crossroads. Her entire left side, from the hip down, was crushed. Hunkeler was paralyzed below her waist with a spinal cord injury at age 21.

"I knew no one in a wheelchair; I had been free as a bird, with so many goals in my life. This moment changed everything," she recalled after the 2007 Marathon. She had barely finished her teenage years. "When I left the hospital a half-year later, I was a woman. I grew up; I learned a lot about myself."

It took Hunkeler another year to become involved in sports, a suggestion from the staff at the rehabilitation center where she trained. First she started swimming, and while she won meets, this did not satisfy her. Wheelchair cycling gave her back the outdoor freedom she missed, providing a rush she had not felt since she was a young girl.

She began racing marathons in the push-rim wheelchair division in 2001, and by September 2006 her career had reached a high point as she approached the final mile of the marathon at the World Championships in Assne, Holland. At the meet, Hunkeler had already won three gold medals, in the 800 meters, 1,500 meters and 5,000 meters races, and two bronze medals, in the 200 meters and 400 meters races.

The finish line in the marathon was up ahead and she still had two competitors to her left. Hunkeler bent her head to her knees to improve the aerodynamics and steered to the right so she would have a clear path to the finish. With her head down, and her chair approaching 30 miles an hour, she did not realize she was veering too far to the right. She slammed into a light pole on the sidewalk and flipped over in her chair.

Her right leg was mangled and she was immediately airlifted off the course. At the hospital, she remembered everybody looking horrified and saying how sorry they were. Hunkeler reacted like any elite athlete would. "It was so strange," she said. "Nobody congratulated me on my medals."

Instead, the doctor somberly told her that her leg was so badly injured she would not be able to position it in the racing wheelchair to compete. Hunkeler had long ago accepted she would never walk again. But she was not going to reinvent herself one more time.

She had two surgeries and was in bed for two months. Ten pins were inserted in her leg so that she could regain her flexibility. It seemed to her so eerily similar to what had happened twelve years before. "You are helpless and you are sad," she said. "But then you recover faster. I know how to handle it. I knew when I give up I am the loser. I knew how it feels to sit in an everyday chair. I knew how long it takes to come back."

Hunkeler began her rehabilitation in the hospital where one goal propelled her through another arduous period: the New York City Marathon.

During her training on the roads of Egolzwil, near Lausanne, she envisioned the start of the Marathon on the Verrazano-Narrows Bridge, far more challenging for wheelchair athletes than runners.

The wheelers must first wait at the starting line for fifteen minutes, growing cold and nervous in their chairs. And then, with no momentum, they must sprint uphill to the apex of the bridge, climbing 160 feet in eight-tenths of a mile. If they stop pumping their arms, they slide back down the hill.

Hunkeler knows her arms are not the only important mechanisms here; the mind is just as powerful, if not more so.

"At home, I always trained on a very heavy hill, too," Hunkeler said. To get her through the training in Altishofen, she would envision herself on the Verrazano-Narrows Bridge and repeat the mantra: "You are in New York now; breathe normally and go up easy."

So this year when she gets to the bridge to begin the race, she reverses locations. "OK," she tells herself, "you are home. You go up the hill now; breathe normally. Go your speed. Focus."

Meanwhile, Amanda McGrory knows she is at a disadvantage

on the bridge because of her weight and her type of paralysis. She is 4-foot-7 and 85 pounds, and she was afflicted at age five with transverse myelitis, an inflammation of the spinal cord that left her paralyzed from the abdominal muscles down. That puts her in classification T–53; Hunkeler, who weighs 20 pounds more, is classified in T–54, meaning her muscles are functional from the waist up. Physics rewards the heavier athletes on the downhill portion, but McGrory compensates in hill climbing with her 5-foot-6-inch wingspan and her lighter weight.

Crouched in the chair, she uses short, powerful strokes to push the inner rings (or rims) of the wheels with her gloved hands. The gloves are white, made from a moldable rubber material that creates friction when they come in contact with the ring. Just like the runners storming up the incline at the beginning of the race, McGrory and her competitors feel the burn. But they feel it in the triceps and not the quadriceps.

The women top out at 11 miles an hour on the crest of the bridge, then come flying down the hill, off the bridge and into Bay Ridge, Brooklyn. The elite men and women wheelchair racers start at the same time—9:05 a.m., a half hour before the elite women runners and 65 minutes before the elite men and the masses. The race for the wheelers lasts a little more than 90 minutes and, because of their speeds and early starts, the elites do not experience the same intense crowds as the amateur runners or even the elite runners. Due to their speed and their noise-muffling helmets, they rarely register festivities or the crowd commotion, turning inward to complete their quest.

In the men's race, the defending champion, Australia's Kurt Fearnley takes an expected lead on his competition thanks to his superior ability to climb hills. But South African Krige Schabort, the 2002 and 2003 champion, catches him on the downhill of the

Verrazano-Narrows Bridge. The pair then speeds onto the five-mile straightaway on Fourth Avenue.

Three weeks earlier, at the Chicago Marathon, Fearnley, 26, and Schabort, 44, raced nearly the entire course together until Fearnley outsprinted him in the end. So at the beginning of Fourth Avenue, Schabort turns to Fearnley and shouts: "OK, let's work together. I'll go with you."

Fearnley responds, "Sure, mate."

But within a half-mile, Schabort realizes he has already expended too much energy on the bridge catching up to his younger competitor. Fearnley realizes it, too, and pulls away from him—for good. Schabort cannot even keep up in his draft.

Kurt Fearnley has been participating in wheelchair racing since he was a teenager; he was born with sacral agenesis, a deformation of the lower spine. Schabort, by contrast, came late to wheelchair sports. Back in 1987, he was a South African soldier fighting in the Angolan War, when a bomb struck him. Both legs had to be amputated; he was 24 years old.

In rehabilitation, he decided to race wheelchairs and began doing so in 1989. At first, he used a regular sitting wheelchair to race in 5K fun runs in South Africa. Now his "ride" is a 76-inch custom racing wheelchair with carbon-fiber wheels.

Unlike runners who can buy a pair of sneakers if their bags are lost en route, wheelchair athletes cannot replace their custom chairs overnight nor can they afford to bring a spare. Twice during the 2007 season, South African superstar Ernst Van Dyk found himself at the mercy of South African Airways' baggage handlers. In July 2007 on his way to a race, Van Dyk flew from his hometown of Stellenbosch, South Africa, through JFK Airport, where he had a connecting flight to Canada. When he arrived in New York, SAA could not locate his chair. Despite his arguments, he said the airline offered him nothing but a 30 percent discount on his next coach trip. Considering Van Dyk had already lost 30 percent of his year's potential income—as well as endorsement money—by not being able to compete, that was no consolation.

Four months later, it happened again. On the eve of the 2007 New York City Marathon, Van Dyk, who won New York in 2005 (and Boston six times), held out a slim hope that the airline would locate his chair. Instead, Van Dyk today sits in the stands as a finish-line spectator and cheerleader trying to hide his disappointment.

This generation of professional wheelchair athletes credits the New York Road Runners and its general counsel Bob Laufer for assembling one of the best fields in the world and for their first-class treatment. But it was not always this way in New York. It took two lawsuits and thirty years of rancor to precipitate the change.

Fred Lebow had been dead set against including wheelchair athletes. He butted heads with Mayor Ed Koch and Dick Traum, a Road Runners board member as well as the founder of the Achilles Track Club for disabled athletes.

"Our stand against wheelchairs in the main event cast us as ogres," Lebow wrote in his 1984 book, *Inside the World of Big-Time Marathoning*. He believed his mission had nothing to do with promoting wheelchair racers. "My job is to develop the sport of foot racing," he wrote. Lebow had also feared that wheelchair racers on the course would compromise the safety of runners.

Bob Hall, a wheelchair athlete from Boston who competed at the Boston Marathon in 1975 and convinced organizers of that race to hold a separate wheeled division, was denied entry to the New York Marathon in 1976. Hall filed a lawsuit that was rejected on a technicality, but Lebow, concerned about the Marathon's image, let him in the race while not recording his time officially. The next year, Hall filed a discrimination complaint to the New York State Division of Human Rights. But in 1982, the State Court of Appeals upheld the right to put on a race just for runners.

Mayor Koch, upset about the bad publicity, threatened to cancel the race unless Lebow included wheelchair athletes. Lebow relented, allowing a couple of applicants but never establishing a separate division. Instead, the race continued its awkward affiliation with wheelchair participants, who felt like second-class citizens. In 1995, there were high winds on the Verrazano, and for safety reasons race organizers were forced to bus the wheelchair athletes so they could start on the Brooklyn side, which meant they would race a shorter distance. The athletes complained angrily.

But the biggest uproar came in 1998, when police stopped wheelchair racers at the Queensboro Bridge for nearly 40 minutes in order to let the elite male runners pass. As a result, nine wheelchair athletes filed suit in July 1999 against the Road Runners, claiming a violation of the Americans with Disabilities Act. In January 2000, the parties settled out of court and Bob Laufer oversaw the establishment of a separate wheelchair division. In 2001, New York finally began offering prize money for push-rim wheelchair racers, for whom there was a total purse of only $10,500 then.

While push-rim wheelers are gaining acceptance in marathons, they are engaged in a controversy with wheelchair athletes who compete riding hand cycles. Many push-rim wheelers do not believe the hand-cycle (or hand-crank) division belongs in a marathon, since the hand-cycle mechanism is analogous to a bicycle. Athletes sit in a recumbent position and spin a hand crank with actual bicycle gears.

The sixty-seven hand-cycle wheelchair participants in the race today are not considered professionals, even if one—Alex Zanardi, the Italian race car driver—competes professionally in another sport. One woman, Sister Mary Gladys, a 75-year-old nun from Connecticut, competes in her twenty-fifth New York City Marathon powering a hand crank because she can no longer run or walk due to arthritis. She has two guides and several friends along the route who hold signs for her as she soaks in hearty cheers.

A full-time, top-level wheelchair professional can earn enough from prize money and endorsements—just over six figures—to make a living. But unlike an elite runner, who usually runs just two marathons a year, plus a handful of smaller races, wheelchair athletes compete as many as twenty times a year.

Hunkeler enjoys a busy life between working, traveling for races and maintaining her long-term relationship with Mark Wolf, an able-bodied hockey player who recently retired as a goalie in the Swedish league. She also has a full-time coach, Andre Fries. She does not think about her disability much.

"The time is going and going, and you learn to handle it with the wheelchair," she said. "Sometimes you want to walk, fit into nice clothes. But I have a boyfriend, a great family. I love my sport. I love to see what I can reach."

Hunkeler's first race back after the 2006 accident came on September 5 at the Osaka World Championships, when she finished second in the 1,500 meters to Canada's Chantal Petitclerc (who is also competing in today's race).

Because Hunkeler had missed nearly a year of competing, when she returned, she pushed herself to the verge of overtraining. "My head wants to do more. I don't like to do anything 50 percent," she said.

Today on the course, Hunkeler does not flash back to any of her accidents. She focuses directly ahead of her so as not to be caught unawares by a pothole or a sharp turn. Occasionally, she allows her mind to wander during the race to her boyfriend and her family. But more often than not, she thinks of the finish line.

Amanda McGrory also sees very little of the New York scenery today, thinking that it must be nice for runners to be able to take in the sights at a slower pace. She has a rather narrow focus. "I look at butts and feet," McGrory will say.

For most of the race today, there are three pairs of feet and backsides: Hunkeler, McGrory and Shelly Woods, 21, of Great Britain. The three decide after the first 5 kilometers that they will work together to share the lead for at least the first half. Although McGrory is finding the pace tougher this year, she is genuinely pleased that Hunkeler has returned healthy, because a full competitive field is the best preparation for the 2008 Beijing Olympics.

"I have ended up finding more opportunities out of being paralyzed," McGrory said. "I never would have gone to an Olympics if I were an able-bodied athlete."

Still, she admits there are those do not understand her sport, nor how hard she must work in twice-daily training sessions on the road, on the treadmill or in the weight room.

"People think I'm in the Special Olympics," McGrory said with a laugh. "They don't realize how competitive it is, that we train just as hard as able-bodied athletes.

"'Oh yeah, wheelchairs,' they say. 'Everybody wins?'"

Not today.

12

BLINTZES OR BUST

Mile 12, Manhattan Avenue, Greenpoint, Brooklyn

In 12 miles, New York City marathoners have already taken a trip around the world without needing a passport. Or even having to leave Brooklyn. They have traveled through pockets of Latin America, Asia and the Middle East. On their right, they now pass McCarren Park, where red, white and blue bunting hangs on the fences as if to advertise a place of all-American dreams. Inside the public park, the red, eight-lane, rubberized track regularly hosts competitive runners from Mexico and Eastern Europe, who join the familiar characters: a much-beloved trainer from Ghana, women selling corn on the cob from steaming cans in shopping carts near Lane 1, Italian ex-boxers, and fashionistas from the newly erected condominium buildings surrounding the park.

There is one country left on the running tour of Brooklyn, on a street trying to change while still remaining true to its Old World sensibilities. Veering left onto Nassau Avenue, the New York City Marathon course runs into Manhattan Avenue, with its brick tenements and mom-and-pop specialty shops. Welcome to Poland. Many awnings and store names are printed in Polish, including signs for two psychics who would probably predict split times for the right price. Sausages dangle in straight rows from the ceilings of butcher stores. Breads as large as beach balls, only oblong, are stacked on metal shelves in bakery windows. A hair salon is busy with bleached blondes chattering breathlessly in Polish.

At the top-rated, charmingly tiny Lomzynianka Restaurant, the borscht is a swirling pool of fuchsia; the veal meatballs, pierogi and stuffed cabbage are all equally authentic and devoured quickly by customers speaking in Polish. But the blintzes, oh the blintzes, must be savored. They come steaming from the sauté pan, thin pancakes lovingly embracing their firm cheese and fruit fillings. Here, crepes, manicotti and enchiladas pale in comparison to their ethnic cousin, the sublime blintz.

Two 10-inch-long blintzes cost $4.25 on Marathon Sunday. Six members of the local Polish Running Club will return following the race to enjoy these specialties. One month later, the owners will have to hike menu prices by 50 to 75 cents in order to afford the rent yet not drive away the Polish customers who come to expect such values.

The rent on Manhattan Avenue, according to Derek Rudnik, the head waiter, has quadrupled since the restaurant opened thirteen years ago. While the place might seem busy with customers he speaks to in Polish, Rudnik says his clientele is 70 percent American, reflecting the growing diversity of the neighborhood. An influx of Asian restaurants—Shanghai-Lee, Erb Everyday Thai Food, Wasabi and, higher up on the avenue, the Garden (a new health food store)—have become alternatives to artery-clogging kielbasa and potato pancakes.

While many Polish-owned businesses are staying in the Greenpoint neighborhood along Manhattan Avenue (although moving to smaller storefronts to save on rent), some Polish-American families are migrating east to the Queens community of Ridgewood. "It's cheaper there," Rudnik said.

For now, Manhattan Avenue remains a colorful pastiche of ethnicity and eccentricity, appropriate for a Brooklyn neighborhood where the most famous native is blond actress and sex symbol Mae West.

Salvatore Puccio is a pizza parlor proprietor from Sicily who has owned Russ Pizza for thirty-seven years. His slices, with sweetly rich tomato sauce, indulge the customer, even if there are few on Marathon Sunday. "I lose business," Puccio said. "There is no parking. The runners come in only to use the bathroom. *Gabinetto*," he said, shaking his head. Puccio wishes he could charge a nickel for every runner asking to use the bathroom.

"All I hear is Flush! Flush! Flush! FLUSH! My lawyer told me to close the bathroom, but I cannot do that."

Puccio decides not to come in until 2 p.m., after the rush, but he tells his cousin to hang a scribbled sign on his awning wishing Alex Zanardi good luck. Zanardi is the Italian Formula One driver who lost both of his legs in a 2001 accident while racing in Germany. He will finish fourth overall today in the hand-cycle wheelchair division, in 1:33:17. With the exception of rooting for Zanardi and Italy's Olympic marathon champion, Stefano Baldini (who will also finish fourth), Puccio is not interested in the race. He is more interested in getting back to business.

He is also the benevolent landlord of the Peter Pan Donut & Pastry Shop down the block. That store has been a neighborhood fixture for fifty-seven years, and Donna and Christos Siafakas have owned the business for fifteen years. On this day, Donna and her staff hand brownies and donuts to the runners. To wash down the pastries, the runners take water bottles handed out by the bank next door. "This is my favorite thing of all time," says Siafakas, who has been offering her goods to the marathoners for the last ten years.

But this year, Siafakas would not be able to forget the scene outside her shop. A foreign female runner in her late thirties suddenly crumples to the street, screaming in pain. Two runners who happen to be doctors stop to help her.

Siafakas will find out later that the woman broke her hip. That one scene of care and cooperation, Siafakas will say, sums up the spirit of the Marathon: "That's why I love it."

On the same side of the block, Irving Feller's store, Manhattan Furrier, is closed on Marathon Sunday. His wife, Selma, is in the hospital. At 81, Feller has owned the store for fifty-six years, ever since Selma gave him the money to buy it.

The front room has furs hung haphazardly; they are mixed with leather jackets from Indian reservations, jewelry, Native American artifacts and his large, colorful geometric-style oil paintings. The backroom is reserved for twenty canvases he paints in a modern style akin to postmodern painters like Kandinsky or Klee. Before Selma grew ill, Feller visited the reservations, trading his furs. Pictures of Feller wearing headdresses are tacked to his wall.

"It used to be all Jewish," he said of the neighborhood. "Now I'm the last of the Mohicans. Where did all the Jews go?"

Feller stands out on this block because he is quite a bit older than many emerging Greenpoint artists. During World War II, he worked as a graphic artist in France for the U.S. Army, designing posters that warned soldiers about syphilis. When the war ended he attended the Art Students League of New York.

His instructor, Yasso Kuniyoshi, was Japanese. "He used to keep saying, 'Attitude, attitude. Why are you painting?'" Feller recalled. So why is he still painting three-quarters of a century later? "You can't help yourself," Feller said with a grin. "It's a volcano, a feeling inside you that goes boom."

The runners passing by Feller's old-fashioned store today feel a similar life force simmering inside them, ready to spontaneously combust and propel them to the finish line.

Since more than half of the race remains, professional runners are conserving their energy and not looking to make a dramatic move at this point. Paula Radcliffe and Gete Wami are about to complete their self-guided tour of Brooklyn; no elite man breaks away from the pack, even to grab a brownie bite.

Runners pass the 1908 Green Point Savings Bank building, with the Doric columns and Pantheon dome; the bank, which no longer occupies the space, used to be a fixture in the community, well known for offering loans to immigrants. It is now North Fork Bank, rising majestically above its electronics store neighbors.

On their right, Saint Anthony–Saint Alphonsus Roman Catholic Church, with its white spires and bright redbrick front, signals the turn toward Queens. Suddenly, the neighborhood shifts to a surreal industrial landscape. Here, on the banks of the Newtown Creek waterway, the Navy built the *Monitor*, which fought the *Merrimack* during the Civil War in what was the first battle of ironclad ships.

Newtown Creek, though, has had a more ignominious contribution to history. In 1950, it was the site of a massive underground explosion from Exxon Mobil oil refineries, which went undetected until 1978. The spill was estimated then to be larger than the *Exxon Valdez* spill in Alaska. In July 2007, the New York State Attorney's office sued Exxon Mobil to force them to clean up the traces of toxic chemicals left in the water.

Too bad the smell of blintzes does not waft that far.

As the professionals speed along—nearly two boroughs down, three to go—they drink electrolyte replacement fluids from their own specially prepared water bottles and have only their own histories to imagine.

13.1

DETAILS, DETAILS

Mile 13.1, Halfway Mark, on the Pulaski Bridge

A marathoner is obsessed with details. Miles, minutes, split times, weather, calories, aches, pains, blisters, black toenails, heart rate, lactate threshold, sleep hours, ice baths, training partners, races, courses, shoes, energy gel, Gatorade flavor, feelings—it is all log material. Past performance must instruct the future.

Two feet past the seventh light pole of the Pulaski Bridge, on an otherwise unremarkable uphill stretch above the still water of Newtown Creek, sits the midway point of the Marathon. Named after Kazimierz Pulaski, a Polish military commander who fought alongside the colonists in the Revolutionary War and died of his battle wounds in 1779, the bridge connects Brooklyn and Queens. Besides giving runners clear views of the Empire State Building, the Pulaski Bridge offers the race's most important gauge. This is where runners know whether their strategies are working, how well they have integrated their diet and their arduous training, from speed work to hill runs, and how much energy they have left for the second half of the race.

They glance at their watches. Time check. Gut check.

At 10:45 a.m., Paula Radcliffe hits the 13.1-mile halfway mark in 1 hour, 10 minutes and 27 seconds—the fastest half-marathon split in New York women's history. Gete Wami is still a sneaker's length behind her.

If Radcliffe were to replicate that pace for the second half she would break the women's course record of 2:22:31, set by Margaret Okayo of Kenya in 2003. That year, when Deena Kastor was an up-and-coming American marathoner and serving as pacesetter, Okayo ran the first half in 1:12:07.

Radcliffe is her own pacesetter today, and her plan is simple: Run out in front and if anyone makes a move, cover it. Radcliffe figured from personal history that Wami would be the one to follow her pace. And she knows that Wami will not try to make a move until later.

Radcliffe, who has had two years to think about this marathon, has prepared meticulously. Her race-day outfit and accoutrements reflect her fastidious personality. This is a woman who knows how to accessorize.

The sunglasses Radcliffe wears are to prevent tension that is caused by squinting into the sun. Even the smallest bit of tension in the face could filter down to the lower body. The sunglasses also hide her emotion from competitors and help break the dust kicking up from the street and the wind. Radcliffe's mother, Pat, prefers that Radcliffe wear them, because she does not want to see her daughter's eyes involuntarily roll to the back of her head, as they often do.

Radcliffe also wears a strip on her nose to aid her breathing; she has exercise-induced asthma.

Pinned to the right strap of her gold and black midriff tank is a red ribbon. Other elite athletes are wearing black ribbons to memorialize Ryan Shay; Radcliffe is wearing a red ribbon, as per her routine. She has attached one to her racing uniform since 1999 to protest what she believes is the sport's inadequate testing for blood doping, whereby athletes illegally boost the blood's oxygen with erythropoietin (or EPO). Radcliffe famously campaigned against EPO use at the Edmonton world championships in 2001, by holding up a sign, "EPO Cheats Out," to protest Russian runner Olga Yegorova. Yegorova had failed a drug test but was reinstated at the championships due to a mistake in the handling of her test.

Around Radcliffe's neck is the thin gold chain her mother gave her. It sits under an elastic titanium necklace, a product she endorses that is designed to restore equilibrium and improve blood flow.

Radcliffe was one of the first marathoners to wear knee-high compression socks. Hers are skin-colored and they, too, are designed to increase blood flow.

To keep the blood flowing to her fingers, Radcliffe wears gloves. White gloves. She is, after all, the British aristocrat of this race.

Kara Goucher is ready to bow down right now, that's how amazed she is with Radcliffe's dominance, even through this halfway mark. At 29, Goucher is the United States' newest and sweetest distance running star, and she is riding on the back of the women's press truck watching Radcliffe's every step.

Her fawning is endearing but also a bit funny, because Goucher is one reason Radcliffe is dominating to this extent. Five weeks earlier, Goucher shocked her idol when she beat her by nearly two minutes in the Great North Run, the half-marathon in Newcastle, England. Radcliffe does not take to second place very well, even if it was her first race back after the fifteen-month layoff. She privately vowed not to let that happen in New York.

Mary Wittenberg, the New York Road Runners' chief, had invited Goucher, a 10,000 meter bronze medalist at the 2007 World

Championships, to watch today's race from a moving front-row seat. Wittenberg was hoping to inspire Goucher to compete in the Marathon.

"I want to run this so bad," Kara says on the truck. Three months later she will reveal that she plans to run New York, maybe in 2008 or 2009, depending on her Beijing Olympics experience. Until then, she will root for one woman only.

"I really like Paula and I want her to win," Goucher says. "I want to see her come back from having a baby and be the best in the world."

After the race, Goucher will track down Radcliffe's e-mail address. She decides it would not be "dorky" to send a fan letter, but she still rewrites it three times to get it right, telling Radcliffe how much she is inspired by her will.

Goucher gets a response within 30 minutes, with Radcliffe thanking her and encouraging her.

Three months later at the Millrose Games indoor track meet in New York, Goucher wins the women's mile wearing a titanium necklace. Yes, she will admit with a sheepish grin: "I got it because of Paula."

Jelena Prokopcuka is nearly two and a half minutes—about a half-mile—behind the leading women. She calculated before the race that she needed to run 1:12 for the first half in order to stay in contention, but today she runs 1:13:23.

By now she knows that she will not win unless either Radcliffe or Wami gets injured, sick or tired in the last half of the race. And a marathoner knows never to bank on others' misfortune. Besides, Prokopcuka said, that only brings bad karma.

"If you are kind," she said, "you can get extra energy."

She focuses on the challenges next to her: Catherine Ndereba and Lidiya Grigoryeva. A quick check on the hip confirms Jelena is still able to keep pace, that the pain in the first few miles is still present but tolerable.

A professional runner knows the limits of the body as if it were a machine; a sudden expansion of those limits is simply not possible during a race, especially when there is even the slightest of problems.

Prokopcuka knows she does not have the same foot speed as Radcliffe or Wami. Her workouts are calibrated to run close to 2:24 in New York—she ran 2:24:41 to win here in 2005 and 2:25:05 in 2006.

Aleks has control of all these numbers. He takes care of the training log, the workouts and the worries. He has always made sure they coordinate their sleeping schedules to the time zone of their particular marathon. For New York, they went to bed close to 3 a.m. the week before they left to simulate the six-hour time difference. Five weeks before the race, Prokopcuka's twice-a-day workouts in Jurmala began at noon and then again after 6 p.m. One day the first workout was a 22-kilometer tempo run along the picturesque route that skirts gated mansions facing the Gulf of Riga and then onto the eight-foot-wide recreational asphalt path that follows the town's main thoroughfare. The driver of one car tooted the horn in recognition, but for the most part, the couple ran in anonymity beneath tall pine trees, comfortable along the same practice course they have run together for eight years. Aleks grew up in Jurmala, so he has been running along this same main road for more than twenty years.

When they returned to their apartment, Prokopcuka checked her lactate threshold by pricking her finger, much like the blood-sugar check that diabetics perform. The lactate threshold—or the anaerobic threshold—measures the maximum effort in a workout and is a gauge for a runner to know whether he or she is peaking before a big race. Prokopcuka scowled. It was not the level that she would have liked. Her evening workout had to be a little more strenuous.

There was nothing she could do then but eat, so she made her favorite shake: Two raw quail eggs; mashed bananas; a tablespoon of homemade cranberry or strawberry jam. She stirred it with water. Then, Aleks made her lunch: oatmeal with dried fruits and fresh honey from her cousin's bee farm. And green tea. Prokopcuka is not so strictly regulated that she eschews sweets. She had a small piece of candy. In Latvia, it is the custom to give candy and flowers for a birthday. Her thirty-first was a few days earlier, so the apartment was filled with gifts.

Prokopcuka's training had been a little off rhythm the last few months, especially after Aleks's father died in July. They canceled their training trip to Switzerland and had to find a different way to simulate an altitude of 7,000 to 9,000 feet. The Latvian Olympic team had purchased a machine in Australia that simulates high-altitude conditions; it consists of a mask and a tube connected to a generator. Prokopcuka borrowed the machine and wore the mask two hours every day for a month while she sat on a chair in the living room sending e-mails; sometimes, she covered her nose and mouth with it while she slept.

"If Mohammed won't go to the mountain," Aleks said, "we bring the mountain to Mohammed."

As coach, husband, best friend and travel agent, Aleks gladly takes on many roles. When asked why it is that so many husbands seem to coach their wives in this sport, he answered simply.

"Women," Aleks said, "tend to need encouragement more than men."

Prokopcuka agrees. She could not be more grateful. "Aleks and me, it's like one person," she said. "I am a runner, but he is my psychologist inside. For example, before the race, I don't think about competitions; I don't have fear; I can sleep very well. But Aleks cannot sleep, he is nervous all the time. He is like my nerve system."

On this day, Aleks stands with the other husbands who are coaches in the Park Room of Tavern on the Green, the landmark restaurant in Central Park adjacent to the finish line. As with the rest of them, his nerves are going haywire. By the time his wife hits Mile 3, he knows her race for first or even second place—and the World Marathon Majors $500,000 bonus—is likely over. How would she maintain her motivation for the second half?

At 11:15, Hendrick Ramaala crests the Pulaski Bridge with a pack of runners eight across. He has reached the halfway mark in 1:05:45. So have the Kenyans Martin Lel, James Kwambai, William Kipsang and Rodgers Rop. Abderrahim Goumri of Morocco, along with Kenya's Stephen Kiogora and Elias Kemboi and Italy's Ruggero Pertile are one second behind. Stefano Baldini, also of Italy, and Ukraine's Aleksandr Kuzin are one second behind *them*.

Ahead in the pace car, Wittenberg breathes a sigh of relief. Her experiment—dropping pacesetters—has not caused a disaster. All of the top names are still in the race. They are only 11 seconds slower than last year when there were pacesetters.

Unlike flat courses in other cities without five bridges, New York is not the place to come to break a world record. Chicago, London and Berlin are set up for such history-making times. Rop, the Kenyan runner who won the 2002 New York City Marathon, was paid to pace Haile Gebrselassie for 18.6 miles in Berlin on September 30. Gebrselassie's world-record time of 2:04:26 came with pacesetters but no competition in a race that was analogous to a time trial.

Nobody seems likely to run 2:04:26 in New York any time soon. Ethiopia's Tesfaye Jifar set the course record of 2:07:43 in 2001, and he is still the only runner in the history of the race to break 2:08.

Would this slow pace produce a faster second half?

Ramaala is asking himself these very questions. The conversation in his head seems especially loud on the 2,726-foot-long Pulaski Bridge—a type of drawbridge—where there are no fans and no bands, just the pace car, press truck and two motorcycle policemen who have been shouting jokes back and forth during the race.

"I don't have a coach, I don't have a manager, so I have these arguments with myself," Ramaala said. "I tell myself when it's time to go."

Ramaala enjoys the tenor of these arguments and would not trade his career to have a coach. He has his own style, his own stubborn and homespun beliefs that have gotten him this far in his career. Unlike Radcliffe, who takes advantage of the newest technology for her running outfit, Ramaala's personality and his philosophy are wrapped up in the yellow pages of a Johannesburg telephone book, which happen to be inside his shoes.

Ramaala has placed the exact same pair of orthotics in his racing flats since he began his career in 1995, and they are virtually worn to the foam tread by now. Yellow and white strips of electrical tape bind the torn pieces of phone book pages which serve to pad these once-molded shoe inserts. (Dr. Scholl's meets MacGyver.) Ramaala's left leg is a couple centimeters or so shorter than his right leg, and his physical therapist in Johannesburg—who is as unconventional as Ramaala—constructed his orthotics to compensate. Ramaala still swears by them. For a man who grew up without electricity, why should he bother with fancy equipment?

He does wear a watch, as do all the elite runners, and right now, he is concentrating on his second-half tactics, knowing he must remain alert but relaxed for as long as possible. Since this is Ramaala's sixth New York City Marathon, he knows the course intimately, and he understands the so-called relaxation will end in about three miles—once he hits First Avenue in Manhattan. How fast will he get there?

For elite or amateur runners, the slower the first-half pace, the more fat the body burns instead of glycogen, which the body will need later in the race. Marathoners want to run a negative split, meaning their second half will be faster than the first. Only two men in this lead pack and one woman today will run negative splits to finish on the podium.

Harrie Bakst reaches the halfway point in 2:13:50. But Harrie is more interested in another set of numbers—milestones he has printed on the back of his Fred's Team shirt:

2/8—A lump was found on my neck
3/21—Surgery
6/5—33rd & final radiation treatment
11/4—26.2

In the middle of the Pulaski Bridge, a man runs by Harrie and touches him on his shoulder. "Great story," the man says, giving Harrie chills.

Until Mile 12, Pam Rickard faithfully followed the orange balloons that her 3:50 pace leader Andy held on a stick. Then she desperately had to go to the bathroom, and peeled off to find a portable unit located to the side of the course.

Pam would call her sprint to rejoin the group, weaving in and out of the throngs of runners, her "most athletic" experience of the race. By the time she gets to the Pulaski Bridge, she has accelerated beyond her pace group.

She storms to the halfway point in 1:54, passing people left and right, and is amazed at how blissfully free she feels. If Pam were to check her wrist, she would find a freckle; she never wears a watch. She has lost all sense of time, preferring to immerse herself in the moment.

14

BARBIE GOES TO JAIL

Mile 14, Long Island City, Queens

Pam Rickard scampers off the Pulaski Bridge and winds her way into Queens, hitting a three-block stretch of Long Island City that could be a knockoff of chic Williamsburg. Vernon Avenue features an upscale coffee shop, a wine and spirits store, clothing shops and a modish Italian restaurant. Near the end of the block, where funky gives way to familiarity, McReilly's Pub stands as a neighborhood fixture since 1988.

Soon, the course slides into the eerie stillness of the Long Island City industrial park, all but deserted on a Sunday. Inside white and tan brick warehouses are office supply, graphics and printing companies. The Queensboro Bridge looms behind the empty loading docks, giving runners hope that Manhattan—and the promise of inspirational fans and the finish line—will soon welcome them.

One year, though, Long Island City did have a bit of non-race excitement on Marathon Sunday. In the late eighties a drug bust went down on 44th Avenue. Fred Lebow sat in the pace car with the race's communications director, Steve Mendelsohn. They heard over the ham radio that the Drug Enforcement Administration had shut down the neighboring streets for the operation, and those closures happened to be along the Marathon route.

Lebow went ballistic. *Are you people crazy? How dare the government have a drug bust in the middle of my marathon?*

"Mendelsohn!" Lebow shouted. "Call the mayor."

Mendelsohn reached the New York City Police Department, which relayed Lebow's urgent message to Mayor Edward Koch's office: The sting would be overrun by an avalanche of 25,000 people if it were not postponed or completed in less than an hour.

By the time Lebow's pace car got there an hour later, the bust was finished, leaving no trace.

Pam is oblivious to any felonious history in the neighborhood as she continues on at her steady 8:40 pace. She has put that life behind her. Not that she considered herself a felon at first. It took weeks for Pam to lose her feelings of entitlement and willfulness while imprisoned at the Roanoke City Jail.

Pam figured she was a college graduate, a mother of three, a career woman, and a runner who had finished seven marathons—five in less than four hours. She was not a typical foulmouthed felon like many of the women who shared her cellblock.

Frankly, one of the jail's supervisors, Nancy Brown, did not care for Pam's high-maintenance attitude. Nor did the other inmates, who considered Pam prissy and rained expletives down on her. About two sizes smaller than most inmates, with a frame made slimmer by six months of sobriety, Pam asked for a petite size in her prison garb, drawing the nickname, Barbie. She has dark wavy hair, not blond, and a compact frame.

"Barbie goes to jail," the inmates taunted her as she walked around in her blue and white striped jumpsuit.

After the prison door clanged shut on her life, on September 26, 2006, Pam was put in a holding cell alone for the first twenty-four hours, quite possibly the worst of her life. She had a migraine headache so bad she wanted to throw up. She was allowed only Tylenol, a drug that could not begin to alleviate her severe pain. No one cared. She was not allowed any phone calls in those first hours.

She spent that night crying and lying in the fetal position on the cold, flat, metal slab in the cell. Pam told herself she just had to survive her ninety-day sentence. Two weeks later, she was granted the privilege to leave the jail for eight hours a day to work with three other inmates as part of the Trustees program. Pam got to wear an orange jumpsuit as she picked up trash by the side of the road or performed community service projects. One day on the way to a job, she was sitting in the passenger seat of the truck belonging to the supervisor, Nancy Brown, and she casually picked up the newspaper between them. Brown yelled at her for violating her space. Pam was not a passenger on an errand; she was a criminal.

"I actually choked up like a baby. I felt like a little girl who had messed up with her favorite teacher," Pam recalled. "I wasn't mad at her; I was a little afraid of her. It's a frightening environment as it is. It was humbling. I was under her authority. It didn't matter that I hadn't stolen anything or murdered anyone."

One day Pam left the group to use the bathroom without asking permission. Brown yelled at her again. Another day Pam managed to do a bit of shopping while on the work detail, which shocked Brown. The group ended up doing some work at Habitat for Humanity, and Pam spotted a couch that they both admired and wanted to purchase. Pam thought it would be perfect for her basement den. When Pam got back to the jail, she called a friend, who purchased and delivered it before the supervising officer could buy it herself.

"That's Pam," Brown said, shaking her head while speaking in her office eight months after Pam had served her sentence.

"I was so wrong about how I approached that jail time at first," Pam admitted. "I was not humble enough to accept I belonged there."

Pam was detached from every sense of reality, absorbed instead in her minute-to-minute need to endure the indignities of incarceration. Not seeing her children was "brutal," but gradually it allowed her to realize how distant she had already become from them when she was still drinking. "I knew I wasn't a good mom, but nobody was bleeding or going without food, and somehow I was able to shut that out," she said.

Perhaps nobody was bleeding, but Abby especially was purposely disrespecting her authority while her mother was drinking. Abby herself drank in high school, she said, to get back at her mother. "I somehow felt the more I drank—something that would disappoint a normal parent—the less credibility as my mother she would have in my life," she said, "because how could she counsel me or be angry at me for that?"

Pam couldn't. Even worse, Pam would admit she was so wrapped up in her own spin cycle of fear and inebriation that she had no idea Abby had been partying. When Abby later told her, Pam was saddened by yet another example of the painful effects of her addiction. "Abby was a great student and a pretty responsible kid who just acted like everything was OK," Pam recalled. "Or so I thought at the time."

By the time she entered jail, Pam had already begun restoring some credibility within her family, because she was committed to her sobriety. But she did not let her husband, Tom, visit, nor did she want Abby to see her there. The jail did not allow Rachel and Sophie to visit, because they were too young. She communicated by phone and by letters for the first sixty days of her ninety-day sentence. The distance gave her time to examine her life with exercise and prayer.

Pam was always a sweat junkie, and once she cut out alcohol she craved the high she would get from exercise, causing the endorphins to kick in and create a rush of positive energy in her brain. In jail, she would work out for an hour twice a day, even making a deal with another inmate to procure an extra shirt from the laundry. There were twelve steel steps from the jail pod's common lounge area—the one with Jerry Springer blaring on the television—to the balcony. The grated balcony was 20 feet long. Every day she would walk those twelve steps up and the 20 feet across and then go back down the twelve steps to the hooting and hollering of other inmates. At first, they would put chairs in Pam's way to block her path. She veered around them, refusing to be intimidated.

Twelve steps. Pam would later laugh at the coincidence. In many ways, these twelve steps offered an even simpler recovery program than the traditional Alcoholics Anonymous program. This was all about sweat, about pushing her body as fast as she could as if to accelerate the end of her sentence.

Pam did what she could to preserve her sanity in a place that she found terribly unsanitary. In the jail pod that was built to house twenty women and was almost always full to capacity, there was an atmosphere of high-pitched frenzy at all hours. Officers were shining flashlights in her face for bed checks. The food was fattening and nearly inedible. When the inmates were allowed to go to the canteen, she chose cans of tuna and jars of pickles rather than the junk food everyone else ordered.

But Pam eventually found sustenance of a different kind. Some of the inmates made fun of her for her strong faith, but eventually she began to temper their verbal abuse when she started Bible study sessions in her tiny jail cell to pass the time. On Thanksgiving Day, Pam drew a crowd of some fifteen inmates, who overflowed into the corridor.

After two months, she was allowed to go home for three days during the week, serving out her days as a "weekender." She found it gut-wrenching to pop in on a home life that was not really her own anymore. And it was even harder to return to jail, where she was often forced to share a cramped cell with women who had committed drug-related crimes.

In jail, Pam's narrow window looked out onto Campbell Avenue, and she could see the *Roanoke Times*, where she had worked in the advertising department for ten years. But the window could not open. It was as if she were living in a cruel, alternate reality.

"I joked that there was this little hell on Campbell Avenue. Of course, every jail was horrible, but I had never experienced it personally," she recalled. "It was a whole other environment. Aside from not being able to leave, you have to learn how to survive in there. Whenever I hear anything about someone going to the jail, in a movie, on TV, I think of it differently now because of my experience. And I had just a little taste of it.

"You do have to resign yourself to a certain degree to live there and figure out how you're going to adapt. It was very hard for me to get my mind-set to where I was going to adapt. I was very blessed to be able to move my body."

The exercise would ultimately allow her to walk away chastened. It would allow her to run again.

Pam was still months away from beginning her running again when, in jail, she watched the national news on November 5, 2006, and saw the highlights of the New York City Marathon. She saw Jelena Prokopcuka and Marilson Gomes dos Santos of Brazil break the tape and wear the laurel wreaths on the podium. She saw the excitement surrounding Lance Armstrong's first marathon. Pam had run seven marathons, but never New York. She only knew from reputation that it was considered the ultimate marathon to run.

Pam's first trip to New York five months earlier had already planted the idea in her head. She had come for business just as she was taking her first tenuous steps toward sobriety. Needing to find an AA meeting to fulfill her quota of ninety meetings in ninety days, she ended up at a meeting for regulars in the Broadway theater district. She recognized one actor, but rather than feeling intimidated, she felt immediately welcomed by the group. It was a sparkling, early summer day, and she had gone for a run in Central Park. When she went to prison three months later, Pam would remember the exhilaration of running in New York City.

Pam left the Roanoke County jail for good at 6 p.m. on December 31, 2006. She did not tell her family every detail of her experience, sharing only some of the relevant ones. Abby gave her a Barbie doll as a joke. Pam still laughs about it.

In the Rickards' basement, next to the cream-colored couch she bought in jail, is a wall devoted to Pam's running successes, including a beautifully framed front-page *Roanoke Times* article on Pam from 1999. Trophies shine on the shelf even as their faceless running figurines hint at how hollow the victories were at the time. Eventually, they inspired her to start running again in February 2007.

Pam rejoined her local club, where she was once again the female star among men, a position that empowered her. On the weekends, Tom drove her to most of her 5:30 a.m. group workouts. (Pam's driver's license had been suspended indefinitely.)

Pam's probation officer told her she was concerned that training for and running the New York City Marathon seemed like a selfish endeavor. She would have to sign off on a trip out of state. But in September before the Marathon, Pam learned her probation officer had released her four months early from her sentence, and Pam did not need anyone's approval to go to New York.

The trip would be a much-needed vacation for Tom and Pam together. Seeking a budget hotel in Manhattan, Pam thought her choice rather appropriate: the Pod Hotel. They slept on bunk beds in a small room with a common shower down the hall. It was like jail, only with softer blankets on the beds, a flat-screen television on the side and her husband in the bunk below her. She loved how she could push open the full-frame window and see the sunset bouncing off the windows of high-rises in Midtown Manhattan the night before the Marathon. She was back in reality and ready to run.

When Pam dashes by the corner of 44th and 10th avenues in Long Island City today alongside hundreds of other runners, she is drawn to the melodic sounds of an Irish-style button accordion and the sight of an older man with his instrument on an otherwise deserted corner.

White-haired Stanley Rygor, whose face bears few wrinkles except for those caused by his kindly smile, is playing for the runners as he has for the past twenty-three years. But he might as well be playing for his bride of fifty-five years, Kathleen. They met under the spell that Irish music cast upon him. It was 1948, and Rygor had been discharged from the Army. He took the subway from his home in Astoria, Queens, into Manhattan and spotted a long line of boys and girls going up a flight of stairs. The boys and girls were so well behaved (unlike many in his neighborhood, he said) that he decided to see what they were waiting for. It turned out to be a dance. He was Polish, but he immediately felt connected to the Irish tunes and awed by the enthusiasm of these teenagers.

Not long afterward, Rygor went to Tuxedo Hall on 59th Street and Madison Avenue. Kathleen Selvy, age 16 and newly arrived from Ireland, was there. He asked her to dance, and from that night, his passion for Irish music would have a purpose.

Kathleen gave her husband his accordion fifty-two years ago.

"My Button," he said, sighing. "The sound of it has no peer; it beats every other instrument. There is a giant harmonica inside my accordion. I press buttons and I draw."

He performs Irish music every Tuesday night at a pub on the Lower East Side. But the New York City Marathon is his favorite gig.

Rygor looks a hearty decade younger than his age, still showing the muscular frame that allowed him to run the New York City Marathon four times—back in 1978, 1979, 1980 and 1984. His personal best was 4:01:54 in 1980, when he was 54. "I just loved the magic of the Marathon," he said. "It was pure hell but you keep going."

In 1985, he saw an ad in the *Irish Echo* asking for accordion players along the Marathon route, not far from where he lives in Queens.

Every Marathon Sunday he plays from ten in the morning until two, only stopping to eat a sandwich that Kathleen prepares. She sits on a lawn chair she brings from home, listening happily to the familiar concert he plays: Irish jigs, hornpipes, waltzes, reels, marches and anthems. He greets runners from Ireland and runners wearing Notre Dame jerseys and runners from Texas.

Rygor plays until his shoulder burns. He squeezes the accordion, enduring the burning in his shoulder, because that's what the runners do.

"These are the poor guys who need the music, the ones walking and so very unhappy," he said.

During his prime concert hours, the accordion serenades those better-than-average runners, such as Pam Rickard. When she runs by his corner, she is suddenly struck midstride by the breathy sequence of notes from Rygor's accordion. She hears her hymn, "It Is Well with My Soul." She is sure of it. She hums to the rapid beats of her heart, another sign on this day full of epiphanies.

A few days after the race, when told of Pam's moment of recognition, Rygor will confess that he has never heard the hymn "It Is Well with My Soul." Perhaps, he will say charitably, she heard what she wanted to hear in those six seconds?

His own music at times moves him for a different reason on Marathon Sunday. It gives him pause to mourn his son Robert, who died of AIDS thirteen years ago. His sadness only lingers so long, evaporating in the warmth of strangers circulating around him.

Some of the slower runners who have been toiling on the city streets for three hours greet him as an excuse to stop. Others are so overcome by emotion—from the moment, if not the day—that they hug him and pose for pictures with him. They ask him all about his accordion, and thank him for his inspiration. Rygor thanks them for the opportunity to play.

"I would pay a thousand bucks to do that again," he will say later.

15

PUTTING IT ON THE LINE

Mile 15, Queensboro Bridge, Queens to Manhattan

Paula Radcliffe scales a cool, dim cave suspended over the East River between Queens and Manhattan, embracing the solitude. The entrance to the lower level of the Queensboro Bridge, aka the 59th Street Bridge, is shielded from the sun by waffled steel panels erected for ongoing construction. Radcliffe's sunglasses catch any stray rays, completing the eclipse.

In Europe, she has been tracked by the sports paparazzi, her every success and failure (even second-place finishes) deconstructed, her motherhood and its implications debated. Even before she had her baby, Radcliffe's life has always been hectic, between twice-a-day training sessions, appointments with doctors and her massage therapist, interviews, photo shoots, sponsorship commitments and global travel. With an angelic infant bursting to take her first steps, a husband who is manager and Mr. Mom, and a career to revive, she has a lot on her mind.

But from her first step at the start today, the frenzy of her life fades to the background. On the Queensboro Bridge, where no spectators are allowed, she has tuned out every distraction. If she were to glance behind at the buildings in Queens, she would see the sign for the famous Silvercup Studios, where *Sex and the City* and *The Sopranos* were filmed. But Radcliffe looks only ahead, grateful to be out of the limelight and in front of just one television camera for the mile or so she will run on the bridge.

Shielded from the glare of the sun and the clamor of the course, she can hear—for the first and only time all day—the steady breathing of Gete Wami directly behind her. As the women climb the steep hill to the middle of the bridge, Radcliffe uses Wami's footsteps as motivation to forge ahead.

She knows that she is feeling good, as if Simon and Garfunkel wrote "Feelin' Groovy," their famous 59th Street Bridge song, just for her. Paula has not felt this free for two years, so excited to be back on the roads again after her hiatus of injury and pregnancy. She feels as if today is a special occasion, a reunion of sorts.

"Paula," her bib reads, in case anyone needed a reintroduction.

"It's like coming home," Radcliffe will explain. "It's like when you've been away for a while and you come back home to your favorite mug and your favorite chair."

The chair is the black sofa she and her husband, Gary Lough, have at their house in Monte Carlo, the mug for her decaffeinated coffee. Theirs is a simple, almost ascetic runner's lifestyle, spent mostly away from their birthplaces—England for her and for Lough, Ireland. Whether training in Monaco, in the Pyrenees, in Albuquerque, Boulder or Flagstaff—"home is wherever the three of us are," Radcliffe said.

But truly, she feels most at home wherever her sneakers strike. Radcliffe is constantly on a path searching for her next victory, the line that marks the course reflecting her single-minded purpose. It is the journey that makes her whole, the process of preparing and running a race even more fulfilling, it seems, than the feeling of victory at the end. Radcliffe admits she never lets either the satisfaction or the disappointment from a race linger too long. Emotion would decrease efficiency.

"Especially coming into an Olympic year," Radcliffe said, "you just move on to the next target."

Her attitude towards everything is that she wants to get the best out of herself," Lough said. "She works hard; she doesn't take shortcuts. She has a very strong inner belief."

By becoming a mother, Radcliffe fulfilled a dream she had even before she wanted to be a competitive runner. She was 33 when she had Isla. "Had I put it off any longer," she said, "I would have resented my running, and I didn't want to get to the point where I resented my running." She and Lough have discussed having another child after the Beijing Olympics.

Even during pregnancy, Radcliffe kept training and maintained her connection to the sport. At seven months pregnant in November 2006, Radcliffe accompanied Lough to run New York. As the surrogate marathoner in the family, Lough finished in 2:41:51. Afterward, Radcliffe found herself sitting in the hotel room wondering: "How am I going to get back here?"

She ran twice a day through the first five months of her pregnancy—75 minutes in the morning and 30 to 45 minutes in the evening. Following her doctor's orders, she was careful not to let her heart rate exceed 160 beats per minute, as opposed to her usual maximum heart rate of 190 while training. As she drew closer to the delivery and more uncomfortable, Radcliffe ran once a day. She even ran the day before she was to be induced, in hopes of making things go smoother. They did not.

For one of the rare times in her life, Radcliffe pushed herself to her physical limit and was not successful. She encountered a different kind of pain.

"When you run a race, yeah, it hurts, but it's a good hurt. Everything is working positively towards a good result; everything's flowing," she said.

Labor was decidedly not positive. She needed an epidural, because her cervical muscles would not relax.

"It was very stop-stop; everything was blocking," she said. "It was more than painful, just frustrating."

Finally, after twenty-seven hours of labor, Radcliffe delivered Isla on January 17, 2007.

Radcliffe felt wobbly immediately afterward. She ran twelve days later. It was too soon. She developed a stress fracture in her sacrum, the bone at the base of her spine. She could not run for eight weeks and was sentenced to cross-training in the pool. Normally, she said, she would have been terribly depressed. But she had Isla to occupy and delight her.

When Radcliffe finally returned to training, she was so anxious that she suffered an injury to her foot, caused by the sudden impact of the roads after weeks in the pool. When she rested her foot sufficiently, she had only ten weeks to train, with very little mileage base, before New York.

Radcliffe has had almost as many injuries as trophies in her career. From stress fractures to hernias, exercise-induced asthma to anemia to hematomas, she has had it all. Her body is not a temple; it is a hospital.

"Probably if you ask any distance athlete, they will have a similar catalog," Radcliffe said. "When you push your body to the limit, there is a fine line between illness and injury."

Since beginning her career in 1991, Radcliffe has had a love-hate relationship with pain. She has cajoled it, ignored it and embraced it, knowing that ultimately she must endure it if she wants to win. "I like to challenge it, to see how far I can push through it," she said.

Who's winning? "Probably I am, but it's an ongoing battle."

Hendrick Ramaala saw Radcliffe when he was training for the 2004 Athens Olympics at Font-Romeu in the Pyrenees. Her house was the farthest up the mountain, and she would pass Ramaala on the way back from training each day. Ramaala was amazed then, as he still is by Radcliffe.

"Paula has broken the body, she has accepted the hard labor of the sport," Ramaala said, putting her in a category he usually reserves for men. "She's special. She can take our pain. That pain is harsh. Once you have accepted this fight, it becomes part of the enjoyment."

For Radcliffe, running now gives her the same buzz she had when she was a four-year-old, racing to meet her father after one of his runs. "It just feels free," she explained. "It's when things click and I feel well and I feel as though I am running as fast as I can."

She feels the same way whether she's running in the foothills of the Sandia Mountains in Albuquerque, New Mexico, on the soaring trails of the Pyrenees or with her father in the Delamere Forest behind her family home in Cheshire, England. Radcliffe's father, Peter, was a recreational marathoner. Her mother, Pat, was a cross-country coach at a primary school. But the real athletic genes come from her father's side. Radcliffe's grandfather, William, competed as a sprinter in the British army. Her father's great aunt, Charlotte, was an Olympic swimmer who won a silver medal at the 1920 Paris Games as a member of Great Britain's 400 meter freestyle relay.

When Radcliffe was nine, she wanted to race in school competitions and soon joined her first running club. She accompanied her father on his training runs. But she was also pushing to beat her younger brother, Martin, in every game and race. She hated to lose to him or to any boy, not to mention another girl. Even now, she sometimes tries to outrun her husband when he is training her.

"It's nothing personal. I'm just a naturally competitive person," she said. "Whenever Gary says to me I can't do something, I'll do it to prove to him I can."

When Radcliffe set her world record of 2:15:25 at the London Marathon in April 2003, she was paced by two male professional pacesetters from Kenya. One had to drop out early and, as Radcliffe recounted in her autobiography, *Paula: My Story So Far*, she thought of him as "a rival being cut adrift." Even though her other pacesetter had to diverge to the men's finish chute at the end, she wrote how she was "genuinely annoyed that he beat me and finished half a second ahead of me."

Neither Radcliffe nor Lough was pleased that she finished second to the upstart American Kara Goucher on home turf in her first race back from pregnancy—the Great North Run half marathon that starts in Newcastle upon Tyne, England.

"I can usually tell the first couple of miles what is going through her head," Gary said. "I knew after a couple miles that something wasn't right. I was not liking it."

She also discovered that she had re-aggravated an old stress fracture from 1994 in her left foot during that race, but she received treatment and was cleared to train. With five weeks left until New York, she wanted to make every minute and every mile matter. She decided to add about 25 extra miles per week before she started to taper for the race, averaging between 145 and 150 miles per week. "That was my little rebellion," she said. "Usually when I have two workouts a day at that point, I'll do cross-training. I had my fill of cross-training, so I ran more miles."

One evening Radcliffe, excited to make up for lost time, completed all 45 minutes of her extra training session in the middle of a blinding hailstorm.

The thought of racing again consumed her, especially since her first marathon back would be on the same course that gave her a career comeback victory in November 2004. During the Athens Olympics in August 2004 she suffered her most public disaster, which she later realized was likely accelerated by her injuries and treatments preceding the race. Beset by a hematoma in her leg, she had a cortisone shot the week before the Marathon and had to take anti-inflammatory pills. She said those pills upset her stomach to the point where she could not keep food in her body, and she did not have enough fuel for the race. She dropped out at Mile 22 in a daze, completely devastated and depleted.

Afterward, the media questioned Radcliffe's mental resolve. But Road Runners chief Mary Wittenberg, in Athens for the marathons, sent Radcliffe a note of sympathy, saying she sensed she was more injured than she let on. Thus began a friendship that prompted Radcliffe to call eight weeks later and ask to run the New York City Marathon.

In that race, ten weeks after the disaster in Athens, Radcliffe pushed back a challenge from Kenya's Susan Chepkemei in the final 300 meters to beat her by three-hundredths of a second.

"People thought that things would never be the same after Athens," Radcliffe said. "That never crossed my mind."

Her decision to run New York again this year had provoked just as much prerace intrigue. Only she and her husband felt certain she would be ready.

Watching the first 16 miles on television with Radcliffe's parents and the other husband-coaches in Tavern on the Green, Lough likes what he sees. He is happy with her confident stride and the excitement only he can sense from behind her sunglasses. But there are still 10 miles to go and he cannot be certain of victory. Wami is still in tow.

Together, Radcliffe and Wami start rolling downhill on the Queensboro Bridge. The sides of the bridge are clear of construction now, and the iconic Chrysler Building glistens in the sunshine to the left in Midtown Manhattan. The runners will spiral 270 degrees off the bridge and onto First Avenue, where they will run north toward the towering Upper East Side apartment buildings. Peter Radcliffe taught his daughter how to run such a downhill stretch— relaxed, letting the legs fly. Radcliffe picks up speed, anticipating from experience the cheering crowds that await her at the end of the ramp. The fans who line 59th Street are the first in Manhattan to welcome her home after all these months.

A t 10:45 p.m. on the Thursday night before the race, Charlie Walpole and Richie Pinkava sat in their truck on 59th Street just before First Avenue, waiting to paint the town blue.

Walpole and Pinkava do not run. The two 40-something men possess middle-aged bodies more suited to extra-large sweatshirts or hunting jackets than wicking shirts and spandex. Nonetheless they treat those who run the New York City Marathon with detached reverence.

Walpole and Pinkava know each other's thoughts like an old married couple—and by the power vested in the City of New York's Department of Transportation that paired them as partners on the night shift twenty years ago, they might as well be.

Walpole has the sense of humor and the sense of artistry. Pinkava drives the truck. On their Thursday night–to–Friday morning shift before the Marathon, they were to start in Manhattan, proceed to the Bronx and return to Manhattan to spray the glowing blue dashes that mark every mile of the course (except on the bridges). They would finish the Brooklyn and Queens sections the following night.

As part of a usual caravan of eight vehicles, Pinkava always drives and relays information about oncoming traffic. Walpole always sits in a glass cubicle in the back right of the truck which holds a paint drum. He wears a headset to communicate with Pinkava about tracking the line to position the spray nozzle over the street. Walpole sprays on a line of 4-inch-thick dashes that are each about four feet long, while Pinkava drives slowly and steadily. They trade jokes to break up the monotony past midnight.

When Fred Lebow was alive, he would hop in the passenger seat beside Pinkava and shout about how to make turns and re-create the shortcuts (tangents) hugging the corners for runners to follow so they could shave seconds off their time. He would talk and trade jokes and tell them what they were doing wrong. The blue line was his idea after he had taken a wrong turn while running a marathon in Atlanta, where there were no such directional markings.

The Department of Transportation uses 75 gallons of a special color—Marathon Blue—to cover more than 35 miles. Although the Marathon is 26.2 miles, both sides of Fourth Avenue in Brooklyn are used for runners.

His crew paints lines for other city events, "purple for the Gay and Lesbian parade, green for the St. Patrick's Day parade," Walpole recounted.

But Marathon Blue is distinctive, as lush as a Monet sky. The trail blaze may seem unnecessary, considering it would be difficult to lose one's way amidst the dense packs of runners that push through the streets. But the blue line is as much ceremonial as it is functional, connecting boroughs and bridges, participants traveling through the city and the people who keep the Marathon running.

Every Marathon Sunday, Walpole turns on his television in Ozone Park, Queens. "We want to see what the line looks like," he said.

Not Pinkava. "I go hunting," he mumbled. "Bow and arrow."

Walpole loves the Marathon even if he never plans to take one step on his own line. He looks for his own handiwork but knows the importance of the larger image New York projects to the world.

"It shows it's the melting pot," he said. "It's diverse. There are a lot of people out there and everybody comes together. They're all happy. They're all one."

At 11:03 Thursday night, Walpole climbed in the back of the truck that Pinkava had been idling impatiently for a few minutes. The caravan turned onto First Avenue, and Walpole laid down the first strip of Marathon Blue in the crisp, clear night before the crowds descended.

16

BOND OF BROTHERS

Mile 16, First Avenue, 59th Street to 72nd Street

Chicken parmesan sandwiches. That is what Rich Bakst talks about to distract Harrie as they start the leg-burning climb up the Queensboro Bridge. Surrounded by hushed echoes of trudging feet, Rich does not want his brother to think about the hill. And he especially wants Harrie to be caught off guard by the stunning contrast of First Avenue that awaits on the Manhattan side of the bridge.

So, Rich asks, "What are we going to have for dinner after the race?"

The brothers discuss steak but settle on "chicken parm" sandwiches. A couple of French runners overhear their conversation and look at them like they are so very American.

You would prefer coq au vin instead?

Unlike some runners who are starting to lose their resolve and begin walking once they hit the bridge, Harrie feels a boost of energy as he enters the first 30 feet of delicious darkness. That spark intensifies the closer he gets to Manhattan and the ecstatic experience that every New York City marathoner talks about.

Before Harrie and Rich can glimpse the apartment buildings of First Avenue off to the right of the bridge, they can hear the faint beginnings of the fervor. They can see the light and know they are almost there.

And suddenly, Harrie and Rich are accelerating down the 59th Street ramp toward running nirvana, a place where rapturous roars swallow the runners' pounding footsteps whole. When the brothers curl off the ramp and run under the tiled archway, they shoot onto the six-lane street, drawn like a magnet to the electric wall of sound.

Fans stacked four deep and leaning over the sidewalk barriers that line the canyon of apartment buildings unleash high-pitched screams, sound air horns, ring cowbells, and wave signs and foreign flags.

This is the moment when every New York City marathoner, first-timer or long-timer, amateur or professional, becomes a champion.

"You really feel like everybody's there cheering for you," Harrie will say. "You're running this race with 38,000 people, but it's almost like the spotlight is on you."

Harrie blinks back the adoration. Then he is suddenly out of breath, his heart pumping with so much adrenaline he feels as though he is about ready to hyperventilate. As usual, Rich calms him down and steers him to their first stop.

First Avenue is reunion central, the place where recreational runners dash to the sidewalks, lean over the barriers and jump into the arms of their friends and family. Some raise their children in the air, and others strike goofy "I am running the Marathon!" poses with arms up for video posterity. While thousands line the course and spill out of the bars on First Avenue, other fans cheer from rooftops and balconies. Balloons adorn the railings, where the party crowd mixes bagels and cream cheese with mimosas or chips, dip and beer. Brunch on the Upper East Side is not always this raucous.

The discerning New York runners or Marathon veterans tell their friends and family to wait farther up in the 100s on First Avenue, where there are no barricades and the frenzy subsides. This, here, is beautiful bedlam.

Harrie and Rich purposely choose to stop at the most crowded part of First Avenue in front of the Dunkin' Donuts on 65th Street; they used to grab iced coffee here every day before Harrie's radiation treatments. Ellen and Larry Bakst, the brothers' parents, are waiting here today with cameras, long-sleeved T-shirts and their sons' iPods to get them through the final 10 miles. Two blocks away waits Memorial Sloan-Kettering Cancer Center, the only destination Harrie has been thinking about for 16 miles. During his six-week radiation treatment period, Harrie and Rich had to take a taxi the thirty-five blocks from their apartment since Harrie did not have the strength even to walk up First Avenue.

Now Rich hurriedly beckons Harrie back onto the course, since he sees Harrie grabbing his cramping quadriceps during the stop. They weave diagonally through the dense crowds to reach the opposite side of the street where patients and staff from Memorial Sloan-Kettering are cheering.

Harrie searches for one of his radiation therapists, Claire Markham, who is somewhere in the crowd holding a sign of encouragement just for him. It was the least she could do for him. Amid all the patients she sees daily and annually, Markham said Harrie left an indelible impression.

"There is always that one person who emotionally tears you up or, on the flip side, shows you what living really means," Markham said. "He has this fearless faith in himself that kind of rubs off on everyone else."

Markham and a colleague, Jeanette Eason, played music for Harrie during his 45-minute radiation sessions. That song is now on Harrie's iPod: Coldplay's "The Hardest Part."

The lyrics (or at least the way Harrie heard them) immediately touched a chord: "I could feel it go down/Bittersweet, I could taste in my mouth/Silver lining the cloud."

The silver-lining theme is his guiding principle. Harrie amazed his therapists by talking not about his cancer, but about his busy life with classes, his graduation, his new business and his running.

"He never seemed to let the cancer take hold of him," Eason recalled. "Instead it seemed as though it was a challenge he would overcome, no question. The other head and neck patients that he would talk with out in the waiting room seemed to look to him for advice."

But away from the hospital, Harrie did slip into moments of despair. For his type of cancer, chemotherapy has yet to be proven effective. And there is still so much unknown about adenoid cystic carcinoma, which affects approximately 1,000 people in the United States every year. If the cancer returns, it can metastasize, albeit at a slow rate.

While trying not to think the worst, Harrie was confronted with the physical evidence of his vulnerability. The night before his college graduation in May, he saw his hair falling out in the sink. As usual, Rich, his roommate in the tiny Manhattan railroad apartment they had carved into two bedrooms, was not far away.

"During this whole thing, when I was scared out of my mind, he just calmed me down," Harrie said. "He made me think rationally. He put everything into perspective, and he knew how to comfort me. He did everything at the right time, the right way. When everything was going wrong internally for me, he was the medicine for my mental outlook. He couldn't do anything for me physically, but he single-handedly cured me, mentally, through the whole process."

Harrie still keeps his Chloraseptic spray bottle with the label he and Rich made: "Nail Harrie's Uvula." Chloraseptic spray was the only antidote that would enable Harrie to swallow without pain and be able to run during his radiation treatments. They devised a game to see who could hit the flap in the back of Harrie's throat.

Harrie finished his radiation treatments on June 5. The family celebrated with a trip to Israel, where Harrie and Rich dunked their heads and necks into the salty Dead Sea to cleanse their wounds, both real and metaphorical. When they returned, and Harrie's first cancer screen was clean, he began training hard with Rich for the Marathon. This is how Harrie would pay his brother back.

Three weeks into training, Harrie did the West Side Highway run with the Fred's Team group. His training called for 10 miles; the group was doing 14 that day, a distance Harrie had never run. Rich was not able to make the session since he was on call at Mount Sinai Hospital across from Central Park.

"Wouldn't it be amazing if I did 14, and I went back and told him I did 14?" Harrie thought. "He wouldn't expect it a month after radiation."

Harrie ran the 14 miles, but his brother was not surprised. "I don't think Harrie realized how strong he was," Rich said. "There was no doubt in my mind he could run a marathon."

Running this race would redefine the Bakst brothers' already close relationship, just as overcoming cancer together had already changed their separate career paths. Rich had been accepted for a residency in the NYU Medical Center's prestigious dermatology program, but he turned down the opportunity. Rich instead decided to pursue radiation oncology; treating the external no longer interested him.

"I really do want to help people, and I want to help them through a hard time," Rich said. "Radiation oncology is getting people through this awful experience, and it's the same as running a marathon with Harrie.

"It's about going farther than you ever thought you would have to go. You have to go way beyond, to a point where you are uncomfortable."

A couple of weeks before the Marathon, when Harrie spoke to New York University's Sports Business Society—he had been president of the group his senior year—he delivered a similar message. "Cancer taught me to be comfortable with being uncomfortable," he told the undergraduates. "And that is a good lesson in starting your own business."

Within the first few weeks of radiation, Harrie decided not to go to law school; instead, during his radiation treatment he decided to incorporate his sports philanthropy business. He called his company Carnegie Sports Group to honor Andrew Carnegie's work to promote "the business of benevolence." In the five months it took Harrie to train for the Marathon, he had amassed six high-profile clients, including Right to Play, a foundation that offers children from war-torn countries opportunities to participate in sports.

"I felt literally *obligated* to give back, because I realize how lucky I am," he said. "From the time I found out, in the first week of February, to the first week in June, that's extremely lucky to go through it all. It made me want to give back."

Ellen Bakst marveled at how training for the Marathon had such a profound effect on her sons. It even caused them to switch personalities. Harrie was always impulsive, Rich the contemplative one.

"He's got to get something done, and he goes and does it," Ellen said of Harrie. "The surgery is the only way to explain it. His mindset was, 'Get it out.'"

But Rich turned out to be the impulsive one when it came to the Marathon. "There was nothing to think about," Ellen said. "Because Harrie was, although not saying it out loud, wondering, 'Can I do it?' This is the one time Rich said, 'Yes—no ifs, ands or buts.'"

Rich ran 4:05 in 2006. He trained better this year and knew he could run faster, but still, time is immaterial.

"Harrie knows that I can run this marathon fast, and he sees how much I love running," Rich said a week before the race. "The fact that I would be able to give that up, just to run with him, that's what I want to show him. No matter how much I love something, he comes first."

The brothers' bond needs no words today, only a tattoo. Rich and Harrie each shaved a section of their head and neck, in the back under the right ear. That is where the radiation took Harrie's hair. In the bald spot, they have affixed temporary tattoos—the purple and orange Fred's Team logos.

Now as Harrie and Rich run by the hospital, slowing down to shake the hands of volunteers and cancer patients yet somehow missing Markham, Harrie gets teary eyed again. But he does not lose it. He said before the race that his marathon would simply be reaching the hospital on his own power. Only now, it is no longer about a personal finish line. Harrie wants to reach the official one.

Together, Harrie and Rich would raise $6,139, which they donate to Memorial Sloan-Kettering's research for head and neck cancers. Fred's Team runners would contribute $4 million of the $18.5 million raised by the twenty-five charity partners of New York Road Runners for the 2007 race. Team for Kids, the other official charity of the Marathon (operated by the New York Road Runners

Foundation) has 1,200 runners today who would raise $3.6 million to support children's running programs.

A total of 4,950 runners entered through the twenty-five charity partners, not including those runners from overseas or lottery entrants who run for other causes.

Perhaps even more than any celebrity runner or one professional athlete, charity running has profoundly changed the face of marathoning in the United States. Fundraising provides that extra layer of motivation; the selfishness of training is offset by the selflessness of the goal.

In New York, running for a charity also is the easiest way a runner can guarantee a spot in the race considering that more than 80 percent of the lottery applicants get turned away. The New York Road Runners chief, Mary Wittenberg, is aware of the implication that charity entries are creating a pay-to-run image, which is one reason she struggled with the idea for a long time.

"We were the last to the charity party," she acknowledged. "But of the 53,000 entrants, setting aside 4,000 or so does not skew the field."

It was a cancer activist, Paul Nicholls, who finally convinced the Road Runners to change their policy. Nicholls used to be fat and lazy, and he smoked cigarettes when he moved to New York from England in 1999 to work as an advertising executive at Ogilvy & Mather. Then he decided that if he wanted to be a true New Yorker, he had better start running in Central Park. Along the way, he met his wife, lost 67 pounds and, while training for the 2002 New York City Marathon, broke his arm. When he went to the hospital for X-rays, he discovered he had bone cancer, stage 3 multiple myeloma, at age 52.

After having surgery, a bone marrow transplant, chemotherapy and titanium implants, Nicholls told his oncologist he was going to run the 2003 New York Marathon. Nicholls recalled his doctor's reaction, with a bit of British embellishment: "You must be off your trolley!"

But Nicholls's doctor at St. Luke's Roosevelt Hospital said he would run the Marathon with him. Together with fourteen other hospital staff members and patients, they raised $250,000 that went directly to the hospital to help fund the immediate needs of patients' families.

In 2004, Nicholls founded Team Continuum and persuaded the Road Runners to let him be the unofficial test case for a charity program. He also insisted that the Road Runners keep $500 per charity entry from the $2,500 minimum the charity runners raised; that way the Road Runners could help fund its developing programs to promote runners' education and services.

As an Englishman, Nicholls was well versed in charitable practices. Since 1993, the London Marathon has always had the highest number of runners participating for charity among all international marathons—close to 78 percent in 2007. According to Dave Bedford, the London race director, 46.5 million British pounds— about $91.2 million—were raised for charity in the 2006 London Marathon. Londoners, said Bedford, don't ask runners what time they intend to run, but what charity they are running for.

"What this has done, it's made running—dare I say?—less nerdy," Bedford added, having obviously not seen the man participating in a gigantic telephone costume in London.

Even before Wittenberg became president of the Road Runners, her predecessor in the seventies and eighties, Fred Lebow, strongly objected to charities in his races. He was concerned it would take away from funds for the Road Runners organization. But when Lebow became ill with brain cancer in 1990 and was treated at Sloan-Kettering, he was moved by the children who were patients there. He understood the value of funding research, and in 1991 established Fred's Team, which at first was directed solely toward children's cancer research.

While being treated at Sloan-Kettering, Lebow would do laps in the hallways—eleven on his floor, or sixty-seven laps around the roof, equaled a mile—inspiring other patients to join him. He promised himself that if his cancer went into remission, he would run his own race, and in 1992 he and Grete Waitz triumphantly finished the New York City Marathon together.

Waitz became the first captain of Fred's Team in 1991, an honor that became bittersweet in 2005 when she disclosed that she, too, was fighting cancer. She receives checkups at Sloan-Kettering four or five times a year, whenever she flies from her home in Oslo for races. On this day, Fred's Team runners wear plastic bracelets with her name inscribed on them and T-shirts with words announcing they are running for her.

At 54, Waitz's face is still graceful and kind, but more weathered than it should be for a woman who earned worldwide fame by crossing finish lines without showing a struggle. A very private woman, still uncomfortable with the onslaught of attention she receives, Waitz does not want to reveal the type of cancer she is battling. She would rather focus on the fight.

She undergoes biweekly chemotherapy treatments in Oslo, but through the exhausting ordeal, Waitz's eyes remain bright. They are cool, deep pools of blue, a color that seems almost unnatural in its richness, but yet one so reassuringly alive. In her eyes is the reflection of the runner's soul.

Humble yet fiercely confident, focused yet keenly self-aware, Waitz talks about her determination and how it has saved her thus far in a race without a finish line in sight. She continues to work out on an indoor elliptical machine, and she runs short distances outside.

"I am convinced that you can go through a lot more when you are physically fit," she said. "It is both physical and mental. With the athletic background, you think more on the positive side—you can do this."

When she was running marathons, the only mantra she would repeat was: "Just keep going."

Waitz lives by that same mantra today, waving to the fans and patients as she passes Sloan-Kettering in the women's pace car. She may not know her own course now, but her journey is a reassuringly familiar one up First Avenue.

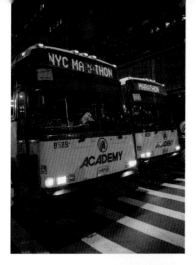

Buses wait in the predawn darkness to transport runners from the New York Public Library in Midtown Manhattan to the starting village in Staten Island. (*Nathan West/New York Road Runners*)

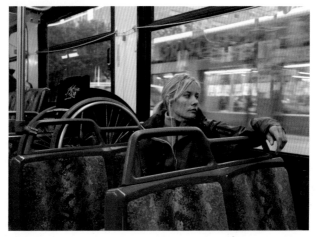

ABOVE: On the ride to the race start, Switzerland's Edith Hunkeler, one of the top women's wheelchair racers, contemplates her long road back from her life's second devastating accident. (*Ed Haas/New York Road Runners*)

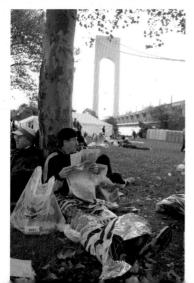

Steve Bryan Vivian, 54, of Ontario, Canada, arrives early at the start village and relaxes before his eleventh New York City Marathon. (*Nathan West/ New York Road Runners*)

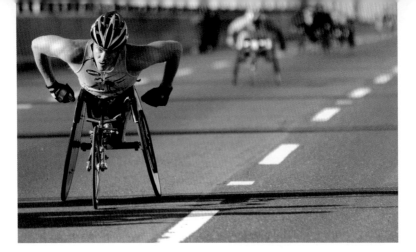

Kurt Fearnley of Australia charges to the front of the elite men's wheelchair pack on the Verrazano-Narrows Bridge and will never look back. Crossing the finish line in 1:33:58, he will repeat as champion. *(Ed Haas/ New York Road Runners)*

A split second after the horn sounds, Paula Radcliffe *(center)* is already a step in front of Gete Wami of Ethiopia *(right)*, and Jelena Prokopcuka of Latvia, the defending women's champion. *(Victah Sailer/PhotoRun)*

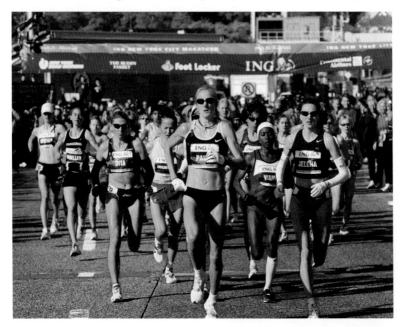

The Verrazano-Narrows Bridge looms in the background as marathoners reach Mile 4, where Our Lady of Angels Catholic Church anchors a corridor of worship on Fourth Avenue in Brooklyn. *(David Berkwitz/New York Road Runners)*

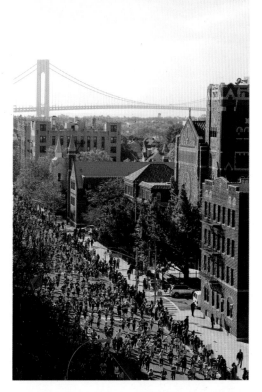

South Africa's Hendrick Ramaala, the 2004 champion, will make several fateful surges during the race, hoping to break up the pack. He takes his first lead on Fourth Avenue in Brooklyn. *(Suzy Allman)*

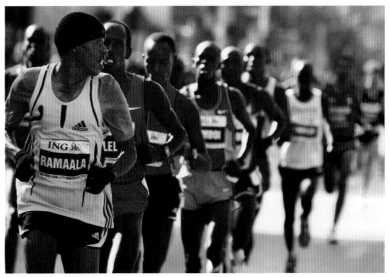

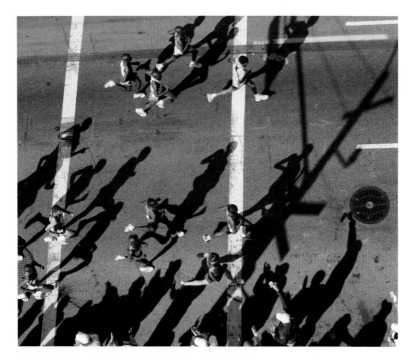

The elite men and their shadows strike a stunning tableau on Fourth Avenue just past eleven a.m., with still more than two-thirds of the race to go. *(James Petrozzello)*

Carmine Santoli, 81, has been a Marathon volunteer for 27 years on his corner of Fourth Avenue and 23rd Street, overseeing operations outside of his apartment. *(James Petrozzello)*

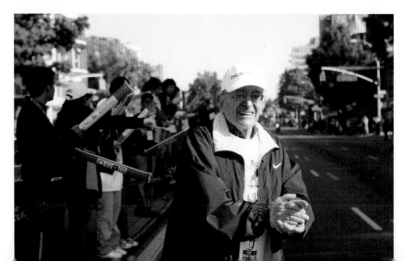

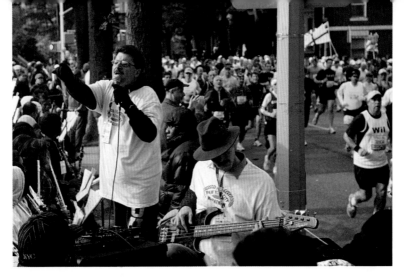

On Marathon Sunday, Louis Maffei, the band director at Bishop Loughlin High School, has led students and alumni in the same tune every year since 1979: the theme from *Rocky,* also known as "Gonna Fly Now." *(James Petrozzello)*

Paula Radcliffe *(left)* and Gete Wami are nearly three minutes ahead of the second pack, at Mile 10 in Williamsburg, Brooklyn, as members of the Hasidic Jewish community go about their day. *(Victah Sailer/New York Road Runners)*

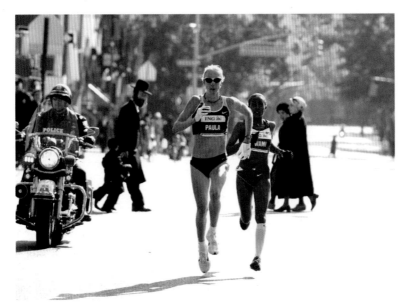

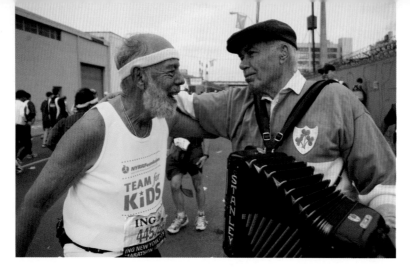

Lawrence Friedman of Houston, Texas *(left)*, stops to thank Stanley Rygor in Long Island City, Queens, for his inspirational accordion playing. *(James Petrozzello)*

Hendrick Ramaala surges up the Queensboro Bridge at Mile 15, flanked by four Kenyan runners: Martin Lel, William Kipseng, Rodgers Rop and Elias Kemboi. Also in the lead pack are Stefano Baldini *(center)*, the 2004 Olympic champion from Italy, and Abderrahim Goumri *(far left)* of Morocco. *(Suzy Allman)*

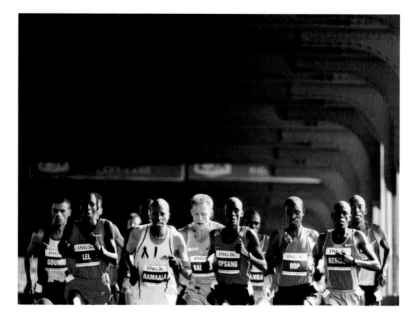

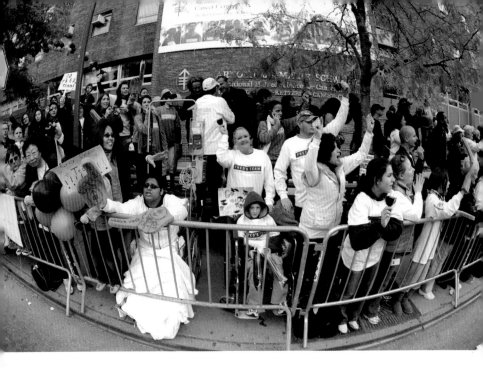

Nurses, patients and friends gather outside Memorial Sloan-Kettering Cancer Center in support of Fred's Team, a charity established by Marathon founder Fred Lebow. *(Jon Simon/New York Road Runners)*

When runners reach the canyon of delirium on First Avenue on Manhattan's Upper East Side, they are greeted by enthusiastic friends, family and bar-hoppers. *(Jon Simon/New York Road Runners)*

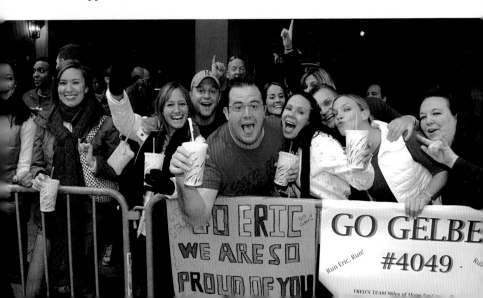

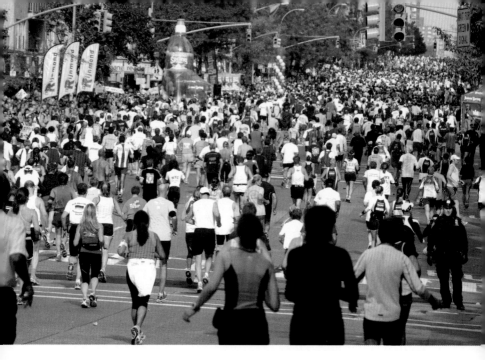

Marathoners flood First Avenue and find inspiration from the fans in the 18th mile. *(Jon Simon/New York Road Runners)*

A fan welcomes runners to the Bronx, just when they need encouragement; runners often hit The Wall around Mile 20. *(Joseph O'Rourke/New York Road Runners)*

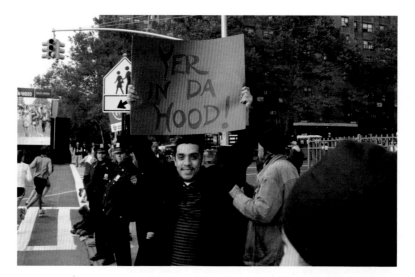

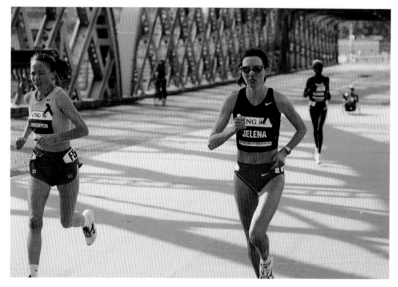

Jelena Prokopcuka *(right)*, carrying a vial of anti-inflammatory liquid for precaution against a stitch in her side, prepares to pass Lidiya Grigoryeva on the Willis Avenue Bridge, continuing their battle for third place. *(Joseph O'Rourke/New York Road Runners)*

Martin Lel *(right)* is a model of calm as he and Abderrahim Goumri break away for the lead in the 22nd mile in Harlem. Hendrick Ramaala (trailing) will sprint to catch the pair, at least momentarily. *(Victah Sailer/Photo-Run)*

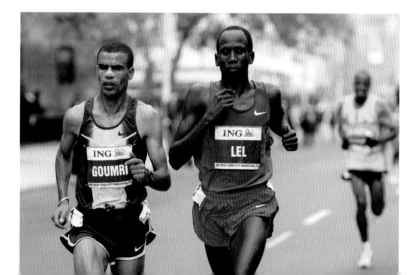

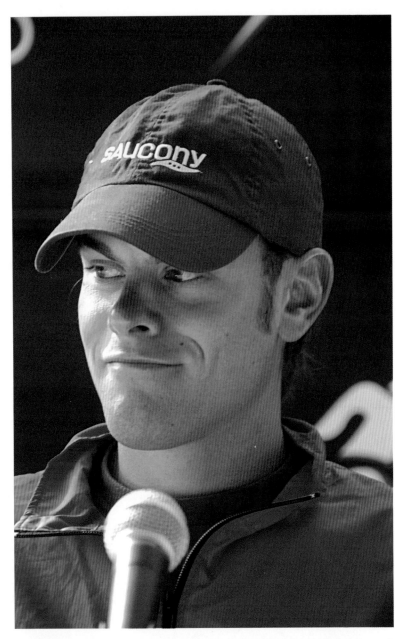

In memoriam: Ryan Shay, at a news conference three days before he suffered a fatal heart attack in Central Park during the United States Olympic Trials on November 3, 2007. *(Ed Haas/New York Road Runners)*

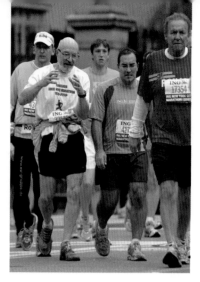

Tucker Andersen *(left)* walking with his new friend, Joseph Shaw, to rest his sore feet before entering Central Park. Andersen has not missed a New York City Marathon in 32 years. *(brightroom)*

RIGHT: New York Police captain John Codiglia, standing on his usual corner of Seventh Avenue and Central Park South, barks jokes and motivation to usher the runners through the final mile. *(Manny Millan)*

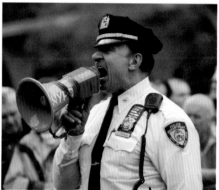

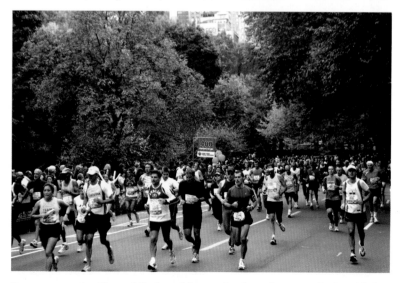

Runners reenter Central Park and know they're going to make it, with less than a quarter mile to go before crossing the finish line. *(Manny Millan)*

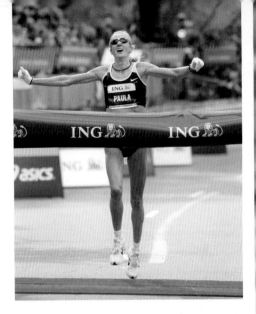

ABOVE: The agony of victory: Paula Radcliffe's reward for setting a brutal pace in her first marathon since giving birth, where she ran out in front for all but 10 seconds of the race. (*Victah Sailer/PhotoRun*)

TOP RIGHT: Jelena Prokopcuka, the two-time defending champion, celebrates her third-place finish, excited to have overcome hip pain during the race and to earn another appearance on the podium in New York. (*Victah Sailer/PhotoRun*)

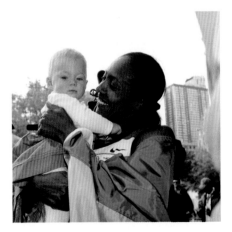

Second-place finisher Gete Wami holds nine-month-old Isla, minutes after losing to Isla's mother, Paula Radcliffe. (*Victah Sailer/PhotoRun*)

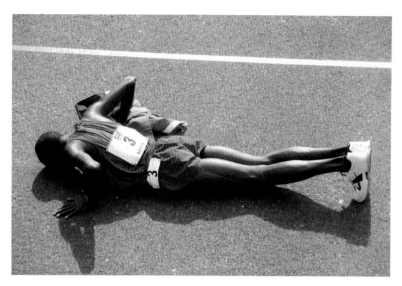

Martin Lel, overcome with emotion after winning his second New York City Marathon, kisses the ground in a marathon ritual. *(Victah Sailer/ PhotoRun)*

The top three men's finishers are genuinely happy for one another. Third-place Hendrick Ramaala *(center)* hugs winner Martin Lel, while second-place finisher, Abderrahim Goumri, congratulates Ramaala. *(Victah Sailer/ PhotoRun)*

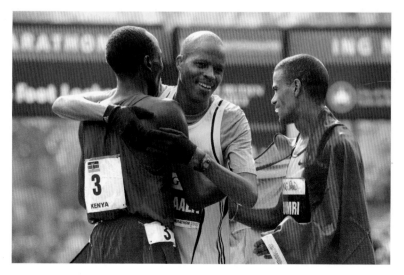

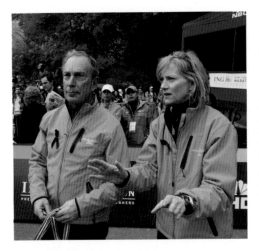

Race director and New York Road Runners chief executive Mary Wittenberg instructs New York City mayor Michael Bloomberg on when to place the medal around Lance Armstrong's neck as the superstar cyclist approaches the finish line. *(Alex Tehrani)*

Pam Rickard, a recovering alcoholic and mother of three from Virginia, trained for the New York City Marathon in the foothills of the Blue Ridge Mountains. *(Josh Meltzer)*

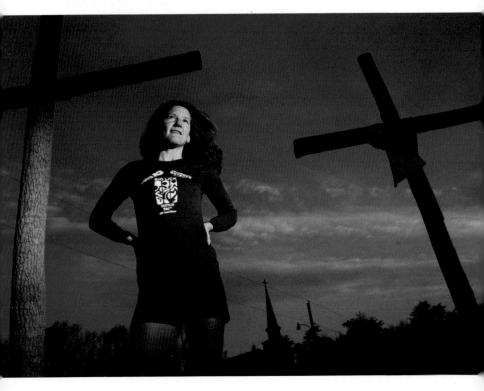

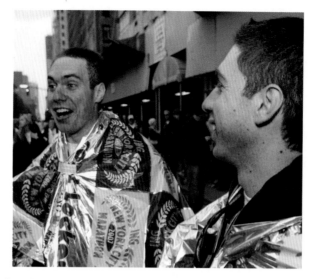

Harrie Bakst *(left)*, who overcame salivary gland cancer just months earlier at age 22, shares the exhilarating moment of finishing his first Marathon with his brother and best friend, Rich, who ran with him the entire way. *(Manny Millan)*

Just before sunset, Cindy Peterson (in hat) crosses the finish line with her friends from Mercury Masters, a New York–based team for women 50 and older. *(brightroom)*

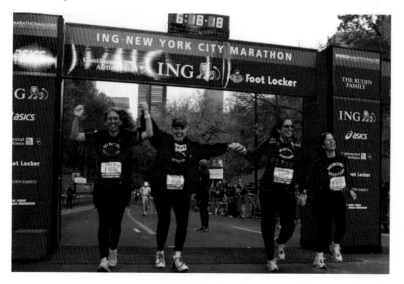

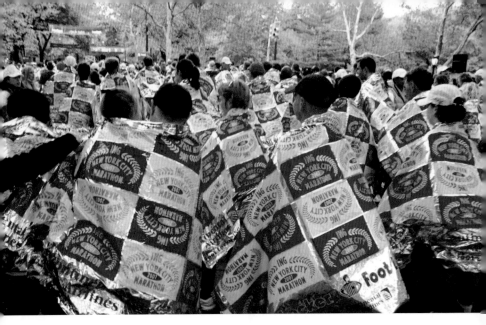

Sea of Mylar: Runners are given heat-insulating wraps after they cross the finish line and make the long, somewhat painful walk to reclaim their baggage and reunite with their friends and family. *(Manny Millan)*

Three friends from Germany proudly show off their souvenirs from their 26.2-mile trip through New York City. *(Manny Millan)*

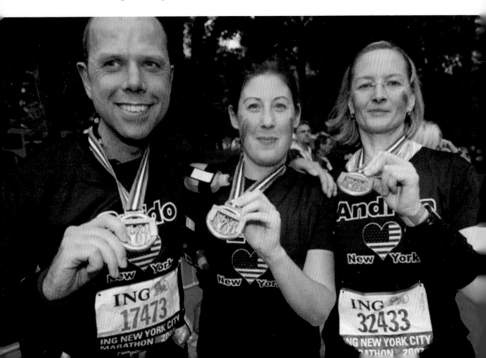

17

ZOO LAKE

Mile 17, First Avenue, 72nd Street to 92nd Street

Hendrick Ramaala is home.

For four years running he has turned First Avenue into his personal play zone, bringing the Marathon to life with his electric grin while creating images of cartoon dust clouds with his bursts of speed. Here is where Ramaala manages to make a very painful sport look fun, even as his intentions are dead serious.

Like every runner—elite or amateur—who emerges from the suspended silence of the Queensboro Bridge into the din of Manhattan, Ramaala cannot help but be jolted by the noise.

"The whole stretch is a lot of energy for me," he will say. "I get it from the crowd. There's a lot of excitement and I guess," he adds later, "it gets to my head."

Ramaala's head seems to be swiveling on a stick as he turns behind him to check the field. He turns to the runners on his left and on his right. He frowns and warns Martin Lel that he is just going to take off. He starts on a dead sprint.

Ramaala drags the lead pack of ten runners past high-rise

apartment buildings and six-floor tenements in the once-German neighborhood of Yorkville. Now lined with drugstore chains, bagel shops, Irish bars and Italian restaurants, the Upper East Side's First Avenue is home to many recent college graduates, who infuse the neighborhood with a lively, if not rowdy, vibe on weekends.

Although it is not yet noon on this Sunday morning, the crowds are spilling onto the sidewalks where a Billy Joel cover band is blasting his greatest hits. The lyrics—"You May Be Right, I May Be Crazy"—seem to be an appropriate theme for the man of the hour: Ramaala.

Stacked with thousands of fans, First Avenue has a seductive power that can cause runners to ride their adrenaline without thinking of the consequences. The way Ramaala approaches it—he either wins the race or loses the race on First Avenue.

"If I don't go now," he thinks today, "I will end up coming in twentieth."

His finished fifth and fourteenth in his first two New York City Marathons—and then figured out the formula. In 2004, Ramaala sprinted Mile 17 on First Avenue in 4:32, drawing two Kenyans with him. The move propelled him to his first major international marathon victory. He also stormed up First Avenue the following year, racing the seventeenth mile in 4:22, but in the end, he lost the race by a single step to Paul Tergat.

"This is where I have always made my impact," Ramaala will say later. "If it ain't broken, don't fix it."

Every male elite marathoner knows Ramaala's reputation.

"In the marathon, he is the show," Italy's Stefano Baldini said. "Sometimes it kills him. But a lot of times, no. I know that when he is in the race, everything is possible."

Athletes come to the race with their own plans ready to counter his aggressive moves on First Avenue.

182

"Ramaala, he is my tough friend," Martin Lel said da[
the race, shaking his head. "He has such high speed. He [
very hard for me."

"Sometimes it's not possible to follow him—he sprints too[
Baldini said, with a similar head shake. "This is a new way to [
about a marathon. I remember twenty years ago, a maratho[
was a regular pace runner. In this moment, everything is differe[
because there are many, many more athletes at the top level and y[
have to do something. Marathons finish with four, five people i[
the pack, and you have to find something new."

Ramaala's solution is to surge at Mile 17 to break up this pack.
So when he goes, Lel has no choice but to follow. So does fellow
Kenyan and 2002 champion Rodgers Rop. For four blocks, the winners of three consecutive New York City Marathons (2002 to 2004)
run three abreast.

At first, they open up a 10 meter lead on the rest of the field. But
Morocco's Abderrahim Goumri, who was told by his coach not to
let Ramaala get too far ahead, makes his way to the back of the lead
pack. James Kwambai, of Kenya, soon follows. Baldini stays out of
the fray and falls into a second pack.

Then the games begin anew. Ramaala pulls back for a few seconds and Lel takes the lead. Then Ramaala snatches it back from
him as the two revert to running fartleks in the middle of the street.
At one point while topping at a speed of close to 14 miles an hour,
Ramaala turns to Lel and holds up his hands, gesticulating, as if he
were a practicing lawyer arguing to a jury of his peers.

Lel understands the message. Ramaala is going to do what he
wants.

"He told me, 'Everything's OK,'" Lel will recall.

For some runners, Ramaala's extraneous movements would
seem to expend energy and create unnecessary lactic acid in his

muscles. Ramaala's agent, John Bicourt, is a little too familiar with those movements.

"I'm going bananas on him," Bicourt said. "For Chrissakes, I tell him, you look around too much. You're telling everyone around you, 'I'm worried.' Hendrick, they're behind you! Just keep going!"

Ramaala does not think he is wasting energy. This is part of his plan.

On the slight downhill slope between markers 17 and 18, Ramaala rips off the fastest mile of the Marathon so far: 4:26.

Ramaala is not a man to follow convention. His training methods back home in Johannesburg offer a window into his performance on First Avenue, a perfect example of his quirkiness, his confidence and his humility.

Ramaala trains for marathons along a 3.5-kilometer makeshift path in the city's largest municipal park, Zoo Lake. For twelve years, he has run in the same direction. Counterclockwise, of course.

In miles, the loop is roughly 2.17, give or take a few steps depending on downed branches, construction and the whim of the restaurant owners who arbitrarily close portions of the public path around their expanding property. To Ramaala, his loop of loping hills, sweeping oak trees and sycamores on uneven terrain represents both the trials and charms of modern South Africa.

"I love my lap," Ramaala said with a grin. "Because it is home."

Zoo Lake Park, built 102 years ago, is in the Saxonwold neighborhood, a five-minute drive from Ramaala's house in the northern suburbs of Johannesburg. The park is relatively small—a little more than 100 acres—but like New York's Central Park, it is the city's most popular and expansive meeting place, offering a diversity of activities. There are monthly art shows, an annual jazz festival, pad-

dleboating, lawn bowling, tennis, cricket, soccer and charity 5 kilometer running races on the weekends. In the late afternoons and
evenings of summer, the park fills with revelers already drinking
to start the weekend; some are excessively raucous. Ramaala trains
through the distractions.

Unlike in Central Park, there is no official running trail here.
So Ramaala and his loyal band of aspiring marathoners create their
own, running three-quarters of the lap along the perimeter of the
park, adjacent to the traffic.

The park opened in 1906, a gift to the city from a mining company. The land was ceded to the city provided it would be open
to both blacks and whites together. Despite a protest in 1958 (following a scandal involving a white woman who was seen dancing to ditties played by a black pennywhistler), the city upheld the
original donor's intent of tolerance. The land totals 200 acres but
a main street divides it into two parts, with the Johannesburg Zoo
across from Zoo Lake. Ramaala has never been to the Johannesburg Zoo.

"A zoo," he said with a chuckle. "I grew up with animals all
around me; why should I want to see them in cages?"

Ramaala's wife, Rodica Moroianu, grew up training in the forests and hills of Romania. When she first saw Zoo Lake, she was
incredulous. "Hendrick, you're crazy to train for a marathon here,
it's not possible to train only on this lap," she told him.

But when she, too, started training there for competitions in
middle distances, she realized how the intimate confines of this
one lap offered the familiar comfort and the precision needed to
measure progress. "When you start calculating, you say, 'I know I
can get in shape for a competition, I only need three weeks,'" she
explained.

"For Hendrick, when he's in good shape, he'll be testing Tuesday, the week before his marathon. If he runs under ten minutes, he knows he can go to New York and run well."

Today, he will easily run 3.5 kilometers on First Avenue in well under 10 minutes.

Baldini trained at Zoo Lake with his national team ten years earlier. He turned up his nose in recollection of the too-small park and the uninspiring locale.

But Zoo Lake is deceptive in its worth to a professional runner. Johannesburg is 5,751 feet above sea level. Unlike altitude training in the pristine Alps or in Boulder, Colorado, where the challenges present themselves as obviously as snow-capped mountains, Zoo Lake makes the runner work harder to find its intrinsic challenges. The gradual hills have small sticks, stones, and razor-sharp palm branches on their dirt and grass paths. The monotony of a twelve-lap training session is the ultimate test of self-discipline for a sport that demands it. The topography of Zoo Lake teaches runners never to relax, suitable practice for a marathon like New York, where potholes and even a loose manhole can lurk virtually anywhere.

Granted, few marathoners train for the race of their lives like Ramaala does. About three-quarters of the way around the park, Ramaala must run with his training group single-file through an outdoor restaurant. They skirt over a path of slippery pebbles, slither around café tables, and then fly down two wooden steps, all while avoiding growling security. The private African-themed restaurant, Moyo, has continued to expand (adding a large gift shop and outdoor stage) without problem, even though it sits on city property.

Ramaala and his group first tried to reason with Moyo's management, in hopes it would not add tables to the outdoor dining area. The owners never made good on their promise to keep the path clear, instead placing the furniture in a way that narrowed the opening for the runners.

Confrontation is often the only way to get results in South Africa, Ramaala explained, and that is a last resort for him. It comes quickly, however, to the youngest member of the running group, Craig Cynkin, who is also the only regular white runner.

His head shaven to look tough, Cynkin is intense, and extreme in his dedication and his mileage. He is 5 foot 7, an earnest 22-year-old college student at the University of Witwatersrand (on a six-year plan) who comes from a warm, modern Orthodox Jewish family. He is the youngest of three siblings, and Cynkin's family does not understand his desire to be a professional runner; his mother and his father, who is a plumber, want him to have a sustainable career.

Cynkin is appreciative of Ramaala's friendship. "I can phone Hendrick any time, and when I speak to him, he's a friend and not a 2:06 marathoner," he said.

Cynkin would do anything to protect Ramaala. One day during a training run a couple of years ago, Moyo's management (who was white) had put up a barricade that blocked the path. Cynkin confronted the black security officers, who were holding knives. After a nasty scuffle, they eventually let the runners pass.

"There's a wall between us and them, and something can flare up at any time," Cynkin said of Moyo's management. "They don't understand. To them, we're just running there, disturbing them."

The restaurant has not been the only point of confrontation in Zoo Lake for Ramaala. After he and his runners survive volatile tempers and loose pebbles at Moyo, they traverse the lake on a brick path before mounting a challenging uphill slope. There they have encountered dog walkers, some more menacing than others.

A few years ago, a white woman let her German shepherd off the leash, and it knocked Ramaala down from behind. Ramaala and Rodica, who was training with him that day, thought it was intentional. "For them, it's fun to see a black man on the ground; they enjoy that more than anything," Rodica said. "We just shouted and told them, 'Wait for next time.'"

One Saturday in 2001, just as Rodica and Hendrick had moved to Johannesburg full-time from France, another white woman was pushing a baby carriage and walking two dogs, a small one and, again, a German shepherd.

"The dog left the owner and was going straight to Hendrick," Rodica recalled. The dog attacked him.

"At that time, we couldn't take any more," Rodica added. "The guys took stones to the dog and defended themselves."

The woman screamed, "You animal, you kill the dog!"

Rodica said the woman then started beating one of the black runners in their group with her dog leash, using it as a whip. Ramaala and Rodica, horrified, came to their runner's defense and retaliated against the woman. They all ended up at the police station for three hours.

The woman, according to Rodica, told unconvincing lies littered with racist accusations; she omitted the part that Rodica, also a white woman, was involved. All charges were dropped.

While confrontations like this are rare at Zoo Lake for the runners, they still have to contend with a lack of respect (or indifference) for their sport. In South Africa, being a marathon runner is not as prestigious as being an ultramarathoner, competing in one or both of the nation's most popular races: the Comrades Marathon—a misnomer since it is actually a 90-kilometer (56-mile) race—and Two Oceans, a 56-kilometer (35-mile) race.

Comrades is South Africa's (and arguably the world's) most famous endurance run. It is broadcast live on national television for an incredible twelve straight hours, after which the race is officially over. Leonid Shvetsov, of Russia, won in 2007, finishing in 5:20:49, a record on the "down course." Established in 1921 by a group of veterans who wished to honor the spirit of those who had endured World War I, the June race traverses five big hills in mountainous regions. And each year, it changes directions. The course takes runners either north or south (up or down), from Durban to Pietmaritzburg, or vice versa.

The 1992 New York City Marathon champion, Willie Mtolo, has been running Comrades since 1994, because it is more attractive to South African sponsors. He has never won, twice finishing second. He can understand Ramaala from both perspectives, as a marathoner and an ultramarathoner. "If you talk about Hendrick, and people say, 'Who's Hendrick?' they don't know him because he hasn't run Comrades and Two Oceans," Mtolo said.

Mtolo also trained in Zoo Lake's park in the early nineties when Ramaala was just beginning his career.

"He was running fun runs—he was just finishing far behind. I didn't even think he would be so good," Mtolo said. "But Hendrick, he was a hard worker. He's a very disciplined person."

Ramaala has gathered his running group mostly by word of mouth; they are young men in their middle twenties from throughout the city. The most promising runner of the group, Zongamele Dyubeni, is a 2:15 marathoner who comes by train from the Soweto slums. Shy and lanky, Zongamele has been both robbed and stabbed on his way to practice, but neither has deterred him.

Cynkin drives himself, in between working at a running store and taking classes.

And then there's Elvis, who arrived at practice one day in a flashy new truck with tricked-out rims and booming stereo, borrowed from a friend to make an impression. The men poked fun at Elvis but still admired the truck for 15 minutes after practice.

Two or three of Ramaala's younger brothers join the practices, one to entertain Alex, Ramaala and Rodica's son, another to time speed workouts and another who just runs for fitness. No matter how long their commute, the runners are always on time for both the 8 a.m. and the 5 p.m. sessions. They place their bags and extra clothing in Ramaala's blue Nissan truck, flex their limbs and head to the corner of the park across from the zoo where the lap officially begins and ends. The smell of eucalyptus from the large tree near the end of the uphill at least refreshes the lungs from the exhaust from the oncoming traffic next to the curb.

As the guys finish their hour-plus workouts, they regroup and high-five each other with their secret handshake of initiation: slap sweaty palms and shake hands with a loose grip ("because we're tired after running," Ramaala explained) and then snap thumbs. It is a ritual extended to everybody, from the casual runner joining the group, including a few slow women, to those who are watching the practice. "Howzit?" they say in greeting, slang in Johannesburg for "How's it going?"

Then, the sunset stretching session turns into a men's club meeting that lasts no less than 20 minutes, even if they had only just seen each other that morning. The runners stretch their limbs on a tree beside the gravel parking lot, taking turns on the old yoga mat that Ramaala keeps rolled up in the back of his truck.

They talk about upcoming races and make fun of each other, speaking in English mostly, since the runners represent nearly every tribe from South Africa. Rodica always comes to the evening session, though in the fall of 2007 she has stopped running because she is five months pregnant. She times the laps and hopes the guys' chat session will not last until midnight. She has dinner still to put on the table.

Quite frequently, Ramaala and Rodica drive one or two runners home to ensure their safety in crime-ridden Johannesburg. Though this often adds 40 extra minutes to their travel time, they do it without complaint and with Alex sleeping in the back of the truck. When they return home, they wave to the armed guard on the street and check to make sure no one is lurking behind the truck as they open the double security gates.

Carjacking and kidnapping are two of the more pervasive crimes in Johannesburg, and Ramaala and Rodica are always on alert. Rodica joked that when people see her alone with their son, Alex (who likes to call his skin color brown), they might think she kidnapped him.

To Rodica and to Ramaala, skin color has never been important. They met on New Year's Eve at a race in Brazil in 1998 and Rodica could only speak a few words of English. Ramaala did not know the languages she spoke, Romanian and French (since she was competing for France at the time). Their conversations were short at first.

"Everything was 'Good, good,' " Ramaala said, smiling.

And it was. They connected instantly. They never had an official marriage ceremony, Rodica explained, as it would have been too difficult for both families to travel for one. Neither runner cares for formalities; their partnership is simply understood.

Rodica is a steadying force for Ramaala, possessing a sharp sense of humor and an easy generosity. Like Ramaala, she does not suffer fools. They both grew up without many luxuries and under strict authority—from which they sought to get away. Ramaala's mother and father, who still live in his northern village of GaMolepo, quickly accepted Rodica.

"They love her, because she made an effort to get to know them," Ramaala said.

He and Rodica share a benevolent spirit. Ramaala quietly supports the promising runners in his group, helping to fund their trips to local races as well as their education. He provides shoes when necessary, but he's careful not to let runners take advantage of him.

Rodica helps Ramaala practice strength exercises at home, as he performs resistance training not with weights, but with the materials they have: walls, floors and the physical support of each other to bolster the body's core muscles. Ramaala occasionally takes an iron supplement, although he says he eschews anti-inflammatory pills or drugs of any kind.

Rodica prepares hearty Romanian-style meals for Ramaala and cooks for team parties. She learned how to bake kosher cakes for her son's birthday (many of his classmates at his private school are from Orthodox Jewish families) and also prepares nonkosher barbecues, such as the one at Zoo Lake after Ramaala won the New York City Marathon in 2004.

Ramaala has won shorter races since then (a half-marathon, a 10,000 meters) but has not won a marathon. He never stops believing he can. He knows how lucky he is that he can coach himself and share his good fortune with the people he loves.

"I eat well, my wife cooks good. I live well; I rest well," Ramaala said. "I've got a good training group; the guys love each other. They are the best guys. It may be small," he added of Zoo Lake, "but it is the best place."

The sight of Ramaala running with abandon today on First Avenue, testing and taunting the pack, stretching his own limits while daring the distance of the marathon, makes it clear that training, as much as memory, has enabled him to succeed here. He is desperate to seize this moment, just as he has in the past; only now, Ramaala hopes he can sustain it.

His surges have helped thin the lead pack from ten to five runners, but Lel, Rop, Goumri and Kwambai are showing no signs of fatigue. By the nineteenth mile, not coincidentally when the crowds also begin to thin, Ramaala will ease off the pace and share the lead, preserving whatever energy he has not left out on the street he loves.

18

KINGS OF QUIRK

Mile 18, First Avenue, 92nd Street to 112th Street

An army of bobbing heads marches north into the rolling expanse of First Avenue, traffic in Technicolor filling all six lanes. Surveying the scene, runners feel the power of achievement—such a crazy, communal effort.

One fan on the sidewalk jumps up and down holding a sign, "Run Forrest Run."

If Tom Hanks can run across the country, then how hard is it to make it to Central Park from here? Logic might be getting a little fuzzy at this point.

The sun starts to hide behind the clouds, and the cool air whistles through the runners' wicking jerseys. The course is still heading in the opposite direction of the finish line.

Runners look ahead and look around. Some turn back to see how far they've come. But they absolutely must look down at this point. For by 1:30 in the afternoon, when runners on an 11-minute-mile pace reach Mile Marker 18, First Avenue has turned into a detritus danger zone. The street is littered with paper cups, green sponges, empty gel packets and, worst of all, banana peels—a bad joke just begging to be enacted.

Some spectators think they are funny, too, reading names off runners' shirts and cleverly adding their own comments from the peanut gallery. Albert Belman, a 39-year-old New Yorker working in Hong Kong, has written Go Albert Go on the front of his jersey for his first marathon experience. He is dragging.

One well-intentioned fan shouts to him: "It doesn't say, Walk, Albert, Walk. So get going!"

Albert does not bother rolling his eyes; he gets going.

As the herds continue to trudge north, another runner's shirt stands out. It reads like a challenge:

Finisher
Every New York City Marathon, 1976–????

And beneath those words, inside the borders of a road sign: No Age Limit.

Tucker Andersen is 65 and running his thirty-second consecutive New York City Marathon. He made these shirts in XL, for himself and for 64-year-old Dave Obelkevich, the only other person to have run every New York City Marathon since 1976—the inception of the five-borough race. They are known as streakers. And, yes, they do wear clothes when they run.

Marathoners are an obsessive bunch; some would say eccentric. These two men take both qualities to an endearing extreme, leading a dedicated collection of New Yorkers who make it their mission to run the city's Marathon every year. Some of the streakers include David Laurance, a 55-year-old podiatrist, who has run every race since 1977; Jillian Lazaridis, a 62-year-old educator, who has run twenty-five consecutive years; and Billie Moten, a 70-year-old nurse and a fixture in weekly Central Park races. She has run the New York City Marathon twenty-two years straight, plus five previous years. At Fort Wadsworth this morning, Moten reveals the secret race day breakfast that keeps her streak alive. "I eat a salad," she says.

The New York Road Runners honors such eccentricity, offering guaranteed entries to anyone who has completed the race fifteen years in a row. But of all the runners who have earned such a privilege, Tucker Andersen, a man with a medium build and salt-and-pepper beard who runs in his wire-rim aviator glasses, could be crowned the King of Quirk. Besides having run thirty-two consecutive marathons, he has also not missed a day of running since February 6, 1992, going at least one mile a day.

"After the first six months," Andersen explained, "I became obsessive over running."

You don't say?

"I am an obsessive-compulsive, and this is a positive addiction and not a negative addiction," he added, as if confessing to a virtual meeting of Runners Anonymous.

Andersen has run while trying to pass kidney stones—twice. The second time he was in so much agony, he just ran up and back on his quarter-mile driveway in Connecticut, two times, in case he collapsed and had to go to the hospital before he was ready. "That actually helped pass the kidney stone," he said.

Andersen has run with ten stitches in a broken pinky toe (from getting caught in a gravel divider this past summer), and he ran a marathon with two broken ribs. His doctor, himself a marathoner, cleared him.

Maybe there is something about cracked ribs that tests the mettle of streakers. Dave Obelkevich ran in 2000 with a cracked sixth rib.

"A month before the race, I took a spill on a curve and broke a rib," Obelkevich recalled. "Until the day before, I couldn't run a 10-minute pace and suddenly that day, it felt quite a bit better."

He ran a 9 minute, 25 second pace for a 4:07 marathon. Obelkevich admitted that it took him another month before he could run again. "I couldn't laugh or cough without pain."

Whenever Obelkevich even thinks about pulling out, he remembers the 1975 New York City Marathon, which was then run completely in Central Park. He had no trouble finishing in 1974 (in 4:20:27), despite the sweltering heat. In 1975, though, Obelkevich got dizzy three miles from the finish and realized he would not break his 1974 time. He flagged race director Fred Lebow and asked for a ride in the X1–9 Fiat pace car—which only had room for the driver and the passenger.

"I figured, there's no point in finishing if I can't beat my time," Obelkevich said.

But soon after he got in the car, he realized something felt wrong about hitchhiking to the finish with the race director; it was the ultimate cop-out. Had Obelkevich completed that race, his streak today would be thirty-four years long, two more than Andersen's.

Soon after that 1975 race, Obelkevich made a resolution: "From now on, doing New York is nonnegotiable. I could have two broken legs and I will still run."

He ran his fastest Marathon in 1982, in 2:40:34. Today, Obelkevich passes the eighteenth mile on First Avenue about 50 minutes before Andersen. Obelkevich does not realize it, but he is actually slowing down. He has picked up a new friend at the beginning of First Avenue and is deep in conversation. Obelkevich wears the 1976–???? New York City Marathon shirt Andersen made for the two of them. But it is his shorts, which bear the colors of the South African flag, that attract the attention of a runner from Canada.

The man comes up from behind Obelkevich and says enthusiastically, "Did you run Comrades?"

Obelkevich's shorts are a memento from the famous ultra-marathon in South Africa, the Comrades Marathon. The Canadian man (Obelkevich will not remember his name) had a friend who ran it eleven times. Obelkevich has run Comrades in South Africa six times. "I want to run that race ten times because then they give you a bib number for life," he tells his new running buddy.

Now that he is retired, after teaching music in the city schools for twenty-eight years (he still plays violin in a chamber music ensemble), Obelkevich enjoys focusing on the longer distances.

"I've done 150 ultra-marathons," he will explain later. New York marks his 69th marathon, with only arthritis beginning to develop in his knees.

For the past few months, Andersen has been suffering from painful plantar fasciitis. This is why he is wearing grayish Nike sneakers that appear as if they have survived a fire, a dust storm and the entire Paleolithic era.

"They have over five hundred miles," he says, explaining that he keeps the mileage for every pair of sneakers on a separate log. He is speaking without breathing too hard as he approaches the downhill slope of First Avenue near 86th Street. "I only wear them for the marathon now. They're perfect shoes, because I have a lot of foot problems. I've worn them six years."

Not intending to shoot for a personal best but only running to finish, Andersen has also picked up a new friend today: Joseph Shaw, 37, from Boston.

They met at Mile 8 when the three courses merged as one, right after Andersen slowed down to a walk so he could wait for a reporter for the local NBC affiliate, *Runner's World* editor David Willey, to interview him. When Andersen told Shaw his streaker history, his new best friend was awestruck. Joseph decided to attach himself to Andersen's hip for the rest of the race.

"He's been dragging me through the last 10 miles," Joseph says between breaths on First Avenue. He reports that he is celebrating the recent birth of his daughter in this race. "Tucker's a great inspiration, because I want to be able to do it in twenty years with my daughter."

Joseph has run three Boston Marathons, sidestepping the qualifying time in his hometown since he works for John Hancock, a race sponsor. With no solicitation, his personal opinion is that Boston does not compare to New York. "I've never seen crowds like this or so many runners," he says. "This is the worst condition I've ever been in but the easiest marathon. Because the crowds are so amazing."

First Avenue is one of Andersen's favorite spots on the Marathon route. He recalls how, in the early years of the race, the crowds were not held back by steel barriers; instead fans spilled out onto the street, allowing the runners only a single-file alley.

"The first few years, it was like a gauntlet running First Avenue," Andersen says, while running.

Before this year's Marathon, Obelkevich recalled that in 1976 the race originally crossed the 59th Street Bridge and went up the path next to the Franklin D. Roosevelt (FDR) Drive along the East River, which included a set of stairs and other unwelcome challenges.

"We were along the river, and instead of seeing enthusiastic crowds, you'd see drunks," he said. "I thought, 'What the hell is going on?' That was the last year we went on the river."

Obelkevich said as much as he enjoys First Avenue and the finish, his favorite part of the race is running alongside people speaking different languages, from different cultures. "The thing that sets New York apart from all the other marathons is that half of the runners are foreigners," he said. "New York is a melting pot."

As a New Yorker, Obelkevich always saw himself as part of the annual Marathon pot. He belongs to the Millrose Athletic Association and lives two miles from the finish line. "I've never thought of not doing it," he said.

Obelkevich may think of the long haul, but unlike some strict streakers, he is not afraid to give himself a day off. His philosophy? "If something bothers me, I don't run," he said. "If it bothers me again, I just don't run. A few years ago, I slipped on a plastic shelf, fractured my navicular bone and couldn't run for five months."

Fortunately, that foot injury immediately followed the Marathon, giving him time to recover for the next year. "I couldn't do all that much," he said. "To maintain my weight, I weighed myself every day—and if I gained a pound, I just ate less."

Oh no, Obelkevich is not obsessive-compulsive.

"He's the calmest, most sane runner," insisted Obelkevich's wife, Lyn Rodriguez. "Some years ago, I asked him if it was all right if we had something for dinner before the Marathon. He said, 'Of course, that's fine.' He doesn't demand anything special, just looks forward to it. The Marathon is something wonderful. For Dave, I think it is a party."

Andersen's wife, Karen, who is in the Galápagos Islands vacationing with their daughter now, does not take such a benevolent stance. "She wishes the obsession were not so strong that I was a streaker," Andersen says, after pausing to answer the question.

For years, Karen had wanted to take a cruise in Alaska, but Andersen would only go if he could run on board or exercise. They found the right ship so that he could run, and they had a wonderful time.

Andersen runs because he feels that he transforms into somebody else on the roads. He becomes an athlete.

In his first New York race, in 1976, he crossed the finish line faster than he expected, 3:38—one of his personal bests. "It went from, 'Hey, I'm going to run the Marathon' to then being part of the spectacle to having spectators cheer for you," he says.

"It changed my self-image. I was always the last one chosen for the baseball team. For me to do something like this, I had gotten myself in shape. Before when I tried to run, I was out of breath for a while. My pulse used to be 80 and now it's 55."

When he started running the New York City Marathon, Andersen worked as a security analyst for Cumberland Associates. He became the firm's chief investment strategist before leaving in 2000 to work as a consultant in his own private investing firm. He was so enthusiastic about how the Marathon made him feel that he began donating to the New York Road Runners. He still sounds giddy to be included.

He works in an office with a breathtaking view of the Empire State Building, sometimes coming in on weekends in a daisy-patterned tie with a green oxford shirt. Andersen looks more like a high school English teacher than a high-powered investor, but he embraces his oddities outside of the office. They give him a distinction that he only has to share with one other runner.

Andersen never met Obelkevich until 2006, when they sat together for a television interview. And then a week before this 2007 race, they met again running in Central Park. They discovered that Andersen's pied-à-terre (he lives in Connecticut and works part-time in the city) is only a few blocks from Obelkevich's Upper West Side apartment. Both have run thirty-two consecutive New York City Marathons, having arrived at this milestone from separate but equally unusual paths.

So who will be the first to give in and replace the question marks on Andersen's T-shirts: 1976–????

"I've got at least five more," Obelkevich said. "There's a healthy competition going on."

(Obelkevich will finish in 4:03:39 today, nearly one hour before Andersen, and he could have broken four hours had he not been chatting.)

There are still eight miles left to go on the course when Andersen is asked to answer his own question. He hesitates before answering: "I take it one year at a time."

19

ON THE PATH OF PIONEERS

*Mile 19, First Avenue, 112th Street to
Willis Avenue Bridge*

Grandmothers storming up First Avenue race against a different clock. Cindy Peterson will turn 68 in a couple of weeks, while her friend and teammate Susan Siderman is 62. They run in the footsteps of pioneers who opened the Marathon to women more than three decades ago. Cindy and Susan are not activists, but they certainly are active. As models for a late-blooming female running generation, one that can be as obsessively passionate as its male counterpart, Cindy and Susan will have run today, between them, a total of sixty-eight marathons all over the world, starting in 1992 for Susan, 1994 for Cindy. They began, of course, in New York.

Today, Susan stops at 101st Street and First Avenue to see her grandson and take a picture, but she does not linger. She wants to break 4 hours and 30 minutes and is just ahead of that pace. She is running pain-free, three months after surgery to relieve her sciatica. Cindy is still three months away from shoulder surgery but is alternating running and walking every other mile to prevent any pain. She is a little less than two hours behind Susan, enjoying the day, talking to friends and her Mercury Masters teammates.

Cindy and Susan were original members of this team for New York–area women age 50 and older. Beginning in 1993, Cindy would drive into Manhattan from her job selling title insurance in central New Jersey to take Tuesday evening running classes with the longtime Road Runners coach Bob Glover and his wife, Shelly. Two years later, Shelly founded the Mercury Masters. The members named their team for the fleet-footed Roman messenger of the gods, often depicted with wings on his feet.

Susan would come into the city to attend the running classes in Central Park after she finished teaching reading and writing at P.S. 21 in Queens. Unlike Cindy, Susan began running at 35 as a way to exercise before her Sunday tennis matches and before carpooling her children to their activities. She started running half-marathons in 1989, and in 1992, after taking the Glovers' classes, she was ready for the full marathon challenge. This was no midlife crisis; it was a way for Susan to reinvent herself.

When Susan was in high school on Long Island, girls were not allowed to play on teams. She did, however, run the relay in the Greek Games for her sorority at the City College of New York.

In 1972, the government passed the federal law known as Title IX, which prohibited gender discrimination in educational institutions, groundbreaking legislation that empowered female athletes for generations to come. Susan's turn to reap the benefits came two decades later; her running has given her new opportunities to compete and to bond with other female athletes.

"This is my answer to Title IX," Susan said. "Some people love to knit. Some people love to play mah-jongg."

Running, she added, makes her feel energized and talented. "And I have wonderful friends."

Today, Susan is the fastest of the twenty-two Mercury Masters. (She will finish in 4:25:24.) "I was always an athlete," she explained. "I tell people all the time that if you can walk a mile without huffing and puffing, that's great. All you need to do is get out there and move. Anybody can run a marathon."

But can they run a marathon under physical and emotional distress? Turns out these older women possess a little of Paula Radcliffe's compulsion when it comes to running with pain.

Cindy ran the 2007 Atlanta Marathon with her right arm in a sling. Two weeks earlier, she had been on a 12-mile training run when she felt something snap in her shoulder, the pain scorching her body. She had a 2.5-inch tear in the muscle in her right shoulder. She attributed the injury to lifting heavy DJ equipment for her company, Singing Cindy DJs. She delayed her surgery so she could run in Atlanta.

"I thought, If I wore a sling, I could endure the pain," she recalled. "It was fine for 12 miles, and then it didn't work anymore."

When her bewildered boyfriend, Ron Vitale, saw her hobble across the finish line that day in Atlanta, she had to explain to him why she kept going:

"You just want to finish it; you train so long," she told Ron. "You never know which one will be your toughest marathon."

Although Cindy and Susan have less wear on their bodies than other runners their age since they started later in life, they still feel its toll. "I don't consider it pain," Susan said. "It's a natural high—it's an accomplishment, something I love."

In 2006, Susan ran New York with two severely pinched nerves. In August 2007, she had an operation for sciatica on both sides of her back. The operation was over in two hours, and the pain left her body almost immediately. She has also had two knee operations, one for a meniscus tear, and on the other knee, arthroscopic surgery to clean cartilage. All of her other pains now are related to osteoarthritis, nothing to do with running.

Only casually did Susan mention that she could have had a far more serious issue. During a pre-operation checkup for the sciatica surgery, her internist discovered she has a mild heart murmur. She kept running, thinking that it was not serious.

Not until a month after the Marathon will Susan have more thorough tests done. And she only bothers because she needs a doctor's approval to run the Rome Marathon in March 2008. Unlike the United States, Italy requires entrants for all races to submit a medical consent form. In December 2007, Susan will have an echocardiogram, showing she has a functional murmur, a harmless sound made by a healthy heart beating strongly. She will breathe a sigh of relief and continue to run as hard as she has for the past sixteen years.

Women are still in the minority today, especially women of Mercury Masters age. Only 12,535 women will finish, compared to 26,072 men. The disparity is due to the large number of male foreign runners, the majority from Italy and France. Only 308 women between the ages of 60 and 69 will finish this race, compared with 1,166 men.

In U.S. marathons during 2007, 40 percent of the people who finished were women, according to Running USA, an enormous jump from the 10.5 percent who finished in 1980.

In a quarter-century of marathons, this dramatic change in gender trends was made possible and inspired by three women, each a former winner of the New York City Marathon, each a pioneer of the sport: Nina Kuscsik, Kathrine Switzer and Grete Waitz.

At 66, Nina Kuscsik, a Long Island nurse, is retired from the barrier-breaking business. She began her athletic career playing recreational basketball with the boys in Huntington, Long Island. She was once a competitive roller skater, speed skater and cyclist—winning New York championships in all sports. "I could do anything I wanted; I didn't feel discriminated against," Kuscsik said.

But competitive running was different in the late 1960s; the Amateur Athletic Union—the governing body of track and field at the time—did not allow women to run in races longer than two miles. Nor could women run officially in races with men. The Amateur Athletic Union and the International Association of Athletics Federations (IAAF), its corresponding international governing body, offered physical (if not sociological) reasons why women could not run longer. Today those seem absurd.

Women were supposed to be fragile; their uterus presumably would fall out if they ran long distances; they could not possibly have the stamina to run 26.2 miles. The 1928 Amsterdam Olympics provided the most damning—and lasting—example of women's frailty, propagated for three subsequent decades.

In 1928, women's track and field was first allowed on the Olympic program. After running the 800-meter race (German Lina Radke set a world record of 2 minutes, 16.8 seconds), the female competitors stumbled, exhausted, into the track's infield. Some had to be given aid, and this was deemed unsightly and unacceptable. As a result, the IAAF banned races longer than 200 meters for women, a ban that lasted improbably until 1960, when the 800 meters was included at the Rome Olympics. The women's marathon would take twenty-four years more to be added to the schedule.

Kuscsik, who had returned to running soon after giving birth to each of her three children, knew better than to believe her gender made her weaker. At 5 foot 5, 114 pounds, with short, wavy black hair flowing behind her as she ran, Kuscsik won the 1970 Cherry

Tree Marathon in the Bronx; because there was no female division, the Millrose Athletic Association members gave Kuscsik their team trophy. She became known as the area's top female runner, and that fall, Fred Lebow heavily publicized her running in the first New York City Marathon in Central Park.

The night before the race, Kuscsik and her Long Island neighbor, Jane Muhrcke, made sandwiches for all 127 runners. Jane's husband, Gary, a firefighter, won the race in 2:31:38. Kuscsik, fighting the flu and the promotional pressure, dropped out after 15 miles.

"I had to finish to show New York that women could," Kuscsik wrote in a 1981 op-ed piece for the *New York Times*. "History records my disappointment."

But history also recorded her triumph. In 1971, Kuscsik lost the New York City Marathon to Beth Bonner in a thrilling duel, with Bonner finishing in a world record time of 2:55:22 and Kuscsik in 2:56:04. They were the first women to break the three-hour barrier in an officially sanctioned race.

Kuscsik had been running the Boston Marathon for four years unofficially before women were actually allowed entry in 1972. She wrote the petition to amend the rules that would authorize the participation of female competitors. That year, Kuscsik was crowned Boston's first official women's winner.

She followed with another groundbreaking victory, this time at the New York City Marathon in October. Just four months after Title IX was passed, the Amateur Athletic Union deemed that in order for women to participate in New York's Marathon, they had to start ten minutes ahead of the men in order to stay out of the men's way in the initial miles. Kuscsik received notification in a letter written by Pat Rico, the woman who was chair of the AAU women's track and field committee. Kuscsik was appalled, thinking the ruling discriminatory and at the very least, patronizing. She circulated a protest letter that every male participant—278—signed. And she organized a sit-in.

When the gun went off to signal the women's race start in Central Park on October 1, 1972, the six women entered in the race promptly sat down, cross-legged, on the starting line. They held up handmade signs: "Hey AAU, This Is 1972, Wake Up." Each of the three signs had a different ending: "The AAU is . . . archaic, unfair, medieval."

When the ten minutes passed, the women started running . . . with the men's race. Kuscsik and Pat Barrett were the only women to finish, with Kuscsik finishing ahead in 3:08:41. The AAU added ten minutes to the women's time, and the two women threatened a lawsuit. The AAU amended their times.

In 1973, Kuscsik won her second straight New York City Marathon. It was September 20, a date that will forever be remembered as a watershed for women. That night Billie Jean King beat Bobby Riggs in the Battle of the Sexes tennis match at the Houston Astrodome.

If anyone in the early days of women's distance running had a similar combination of chutzpah and media savvy as King, it was Kathrine Switzer. She registered for the men-only 1967 Boston Marathon as K. V. Switzer. When her gender was discovered during the race—she was wearing a band above her forehead to keep her hair flowing behind her—the Boston Marathon race director, Jock Semple, ran onto the course and tried to tear the race bib No. 261 off her. The press truck captured the entire scene for posterity. Switzer, who was not tiny at 5 foot 8, 135 pounds, eluded him with the help of her beefy then-boyfriend and continued to the finish line in 4:20:02.

That image, combined with Kuscsik's legislating as a member of track and field committees, changed the course of women's distance running.

Switzer and Kuscsik worked with Lebow in 1972 to found the

world's first women-only road race, the 10K Crazylegs Mini Marathon (named after the miniskirt and the shaving gel maker that sponsored it; stocking company L'eggs later stepped in as sponsor). The race was—and still is—run in Central Park every June.

Switzer then organized a women-only marathon series, the Avon International Running Circuit. At that time, both she and Kuscsik were lobbying to have the women's marathon be included in the Olympics. The distance race was finally added to the program at the 1984 Los Angeles Games.

"It was like getting the vote when men thought that women didn't have the intellectual capability—that it was inappropriate for them to vote," said Switzer, 60.

"Now you're seeing more registered women runners than ever before," she added. "There are masses of women who now realize they have no sense of limitation. They have broken the mental barrier, in terms of their unique capability and stamina. The future holds more for women in the marathon."

Grete Waitz never ran marathons on a crusade—that would not fit her shy nature. Still, by the time she had won the last of nine New York City Marathons in 1988, she had become the world's premier woman distance runner and the blond-haired darling of the city. Before one marathon in New York, a homeless man pushing a shopping cart saw her on the street and cried, "Good luck, Mrs. Waitz!"

Waitz's marathon success began on a lark. By the time she was 23, she was an international star in track and field, having set a world record in the 3,000 meters. She had kept her day job, though, as a high school geography teacher in Oslo, and she considered retiring from track and field in 1978.

But then her husband and coach, Jack, suggested a trip to York. Waitz had never been there, let alone anywhere in the U States. Jack thought it was time she took a long run there, s asked race director Fred Lebow for an entry to the New York (Marathon. Lebow only thought Waitz would make an excelle pacesetter based on her success on the track. He offered her a plai ticket, but with no more money in the budget, he did not offer on to Jack. Waitz refused to come without him. It was not until three days before the race that Jack got his ticket, too.

Waitz never completed a training run longer than 13 miles, but still Jack sensed that his wife was ready for more. He knew her discipline and her toughness, having trained with her and her brothers for nearly five years in the same running club. What neither of them knew then, however, was proper marathon nutrition.

As shocking as her debut would be, what Waitz ate the night before the 1978 New York City Marathon—that is the stuff of legend.

"I had never heard of carbo-loading," Waitz recalled. "I figured this is our first and last time in New York, so we had shrimp cocktail, filet mignon, baked potato and ice cream, plus a bottle of red wine."

Two men who were runners and apparent international track and field followers sat at the table next to them.

"A man came up to me and said, 'Excuse me, are you Grete Waitz?'"

Waitz nodded.

"Are you running tomorrow?" he asked.

She nodded again.

"He looked me up and down," she recalled. "And then he said, 'Good luck.'"

Waitz was understandably dehydrated during the race, although

she did not notice it until she hit Manhattan. "I felt so good, I took the lead and pushed the pace," she said. "I was the first woman on First Avenue, and the crowds there went crazy. They were yelling and screaming. For me, it was like running downhill with a tailwind, I felt like I was flying."

Then, on upper First Avenue, on the way to the Bronx, her race changed abruptly. "It was like someone gave me two winter coats and a backpack," she said.

Waitz was hurting and she was angry, her muscles unaccustomed to the distance, her feet covered in blisters. With no map and no money, finishing was the only way she was going to get back to Jack and tell him just what she thought about marathons.

Wearing bib No. 1173, she set a world record, in 2:32:30. "Who is this blond lady?" she remembered hearing a fan say after she came through the chute at the finish.

Waitz promptly took off her sneakers and threw them at her mild-mannered husband. "I'll never do this stupid thing again," she shouted to Jack in Norwegian.

When Switzer, then working for CBS radio, interviewed her, Waitz was still steaming over the experience.

"I am not a marathoner; I'm a 3,000-meter runner," she said to Switzer.

Waitz soon changed that perception. She started training on longer runs in Norway and was better prepared the next fall for New York. In 1979, she ran five minutes faster and set another world record—2:27:33—becoming the first woman to run under 2:30. Her prerace routine in 1979?

"She and her brother went over to Rockefeller Center and went for a skate," Jack recalled with a laugh. "I was so furious. I said, 'You guys are crazy.'

"Grete hadn't been skating for 15 years. It's not that you'll fall

and get hurt; it's just that you'll get stiff. She's the only marathoner in the world that's been skating the day before setting a world record."

By the mid-eighties in New York, the Marathon was no longer a waltz in the park for Waitz, however.

"I knew that people expected me to win—and that was pressure," she said.

She would have a recurring nightmare that she got lost and could not find the starting line or that she forgot her shorts. "Sitting there on the bus to the start, the last thing you want to do is run the New York City Marathon," she said.

"Why do I put myself through this? You feel the pressure, the expectation you put on yourself, from people back in Norway. Not a comfortable situation. I wish the bus broke down so I never made it to the starting line. I was so sure, though, that if it broke down, I would be mad."

In 1988, at age 35, Waitz won her final New York City Marathon title, in 2:28:07. She would return after two years of injuries to run in 1990, only to finish fourth and soon after announce her retirement. Two years later, she accompanied Lebow in his Marathon run, an experience that only solidified her image as a New York icon.

"Races and cities need heroes, and she certainly was that for New York," said Allan Steinfeld, the race director who succeeded Lebow, and a close friend of Waitz. "She was the reigning queen."

Although he said some critics believe that Waitz never ran against the best competition in New York, Steinfeld denied that: "We didn't stack the field in her favor. Certainly Grete wouldn't have wanted that."

To her résumé she added a 1983 World Championship gold medal in the marathon and an Olympic silver medal in the inaugural 1984 women's marathon, when, beset by back spasms, she finished behind the U.S. legend-in-waiting, Joan Benoit. By the eighties, Waitz's fame exploded in Norway. She started a women's 5-kilometer race in Oslo, which ballooned to 40,000 runners in twenty years. It became too large for her to monitor to her standards, so she disbanded it.

She always preferred the quiet of running on snow in the back streets and woods of Oslo, which she first did as a teenager with her brothers, Jan and Arild. Like their famous sister, each brother has run the New York City Marathon, Jan for twenty-five years—only they get to do it in anonymity. Even now, when signing books or autographs, Waitz is not entirely comfortable with the attention.

The night before the *More* magazine–sponsored marathon and half-marathon in April 2008, a women-only race in Central Park geared toward runners who are 40 and older, Waitz would address a group of participants. "If someone had told me thirty years ago that women would be running marathons like they are today, I would have thought it was science fiction," Waitz would tell her rapt audience.

She did not realize at the peak of her career that she would be the gateway to the future, allowing not only stars like Paula Radcliffe to succeed, but grandmothers like Cindy Peterson and Susan Siderman to thrive.

The well-worn path up First Avenue is about to end in thirteen blocks, and already the course has quieted to a dull hum. The runners pass Thomas Jefferson Park to their right at 114th Street, where young New Yorkers play weekend soccer and baseball games. Housing projects and apartments, hair salons and drugstores are sprinkled on the west side of the street in a neighborhood now known as Spanish Harlem (which used to be Italian). It is still home to a landmark—the original Patsy's Pizza, on the block between 117th and 118th streets. Pasquale Lancieri opened the restaurant in 1933 after training at Lombardi's, the Little Italy restaurant regarded as New York's first pizzeria. This Patsy's is famous for its coal-fired pies and slices—the ultimate New York icon. Tradition dies hard.

A slice right now would actually sit rather like coal in a runner's stomach. But with the toughest stretch of the race ahead, runners must summon energy from somewhere—before their bodies deplete it naturally. They must power their own path.

20

THE WALL

Mile 20, the Bronx

Now the race really begins.

Time for the professionals to go to work. Time for the amateurs to dig in so they can go to work Monday with a medal.

A little more than six miles remain as the course heads into the Bronx and in the opposite direction of the finish line. That unsettling thought prompts an internal debate.

The body—with input from bones, muscles, ligaments—says it is not built to go any farther. The mind, trying desperately to shout over the body's protests, declares it will finish—somehow.

Just past the 20-mile marker for some, or perhaps Mile 22 or Mile 24 for others, the body (of a nonprofessional) has depleted its glycogen stores and starts turning to its fat stores for energy. Neither mind nor body responds instantly during this transition.

"It is like running on a poorer grade of gasoline," said Dave Martin, a professor emeritus of exercise physiology at Georgia State, a regular consultant for USA Track & Field and a marathon historian. He knows The Wall.

The formula for hitting it is simple. Runners store 2,000 calories worth of glycogen in the liver and muscles. And runners burn 100 calories per mile. By Mile 20, therefore, the glycogen should be gone.

Amateur runners know to grab paper cups of Gatorade, and not just water, at stops along the course. Elite runners have their own squirt bottles with special fluid replacement liquids that they mark before the race and grab at designated tables.

And runners have become more sophisticated in their training and understand that getting the body accustomed to storing carbohydrates—before the race and during the race—will delay the advent of The Wall. The more 20-mile runs they complete before the big race, followed by carbo-loading meals, the more the body will be exposed to glycogen depletion and be better prepared to fight its effects.

Every runner knows what The Wall is, and that it is coming, even if they do not know why it happens or where the term comes from. "It's a chicken and egg question," Martin said.

The exhaustion scrambles the mind, and the solution is not to think, but to keep running. And to listen to the growing crowds of fans who take pride in helping runners get past that Wall.

"You're in the Bronx now!" shouts one fan a couple of blocks off the Willis Avenue Bridge, which connects Upper Manhattan at 125th Street to 134th Street in the Bronx.

"We're glad you're back!"

"Thank you for running through—see you next year!"

Runners in the New York City Marathon used to tell a Bronx tale of desolation, a soaring wasteland of wide streets and junk yards with Yankee Stadium rising in the background. Handfuls of fans stood on the sidewalks cheering, but the neighborhood's energy, in direct contrast to First Avenue, reflected the runners' own deflation.

Those images have changed over the past few years. Today the Bronx enthusiasm starts on the Willis Avenue Bridge, where Pat Duffy's New York Scottish Pipe and Drums corps has been playing for five years. Like the other bridges on the course, spectators are not allowed. But Duffy snuck onto the bridge with his bagpipes in 2002. He applied to have his band return and now serenades dragging runners with uplifting tunes including "Yankee Doodle Dandy" and "You're a Grand Old Flag," and because he knows his foreign audience—"La Marseillaise" (the French national anthem), "Muss I Denn" (based on a German folk song) and "Waltzing Matilda" (Australia's best-known folk song).

"I recall the Willis Avenue Bridge being a no-man's-land," said Duffy, 46, a runner himself. "Now, as runners go by, the reception you get is amazing. You see the pumping of the fists and put a smile on their face, which is important especially at that place, which is The Wall."

Not even two blocks after the Willis Avenue Bridge, runners are treated to a large, new soundstage that hosts three hours of continuous live music, from bongo drums and electric guitar to a harp. A jumbotron showing the race live is next to the stage. Down the road on another stage, a DJ makes connections between fans and runners. Residents, relatives and friends shout timely encouragement, wave flags for different countries and hold signs for friends.

Before Central Park became the epicenter of New York's running scene, the Bronx hosted most of the city's races—from the cross-country course in Van Cortlandt Park to the streets around Yankee Stadium. In 1958, a group of forty runners met at Macomb's Dam Park's track in the shadow of the stadium, and they formed the club we now call the New York Road Runners.

In 1969, Fred Lebow ran his first road race in the Bronx, a 5-miler, which consisted of eleven laps around Yankee Stadium. He also ran his first marathon in the Bronx, the 1970 Cherry Tree Marathon. While dodging cars and children who were throwing stones, he decided it was time to put on a marathon in Central Park, where the roads at least could be closed.

When the marathon returned to the Bronx in 1976 for the first five-borough race, it was a token visit. The course crossed over the Willis Avenue Bridge and the runners had to touch a light pole a few feet over the bridge in the Bronx and run back the same way to Manhattan, as if they were scared to linger any longer. (These were the days when the Bronx was burning, although no rioter would dare interrupt the Marathon with the city's police out in force that day.) After people in the Bronx protested that their borough had been snubbed, Marathon director Fred Lebow added one mile of the Bronx to the course in 1977.

The Bronx initially may have been little more than a check on the five-borough list, but it did witness one of the more significant scenes of American distance running.

The 1972 Olympic gold medalist Frank Shorter and the 1975 Boston Marathon champion Bill Rodgers were supposed to have their marathon showdown in 1976 at the Montreal Olympics. Shorter was far stronger in Montreal that July day, winning the silver medal while Rodgers finished fortieth. The two rivals arrived to compete that fall in New York. Shorter came out of curiosity to see whether Lebow could actually get the city to close the streets for the five-borough race, and Rodgers came to make good on his potential.

They spotted each other on the Willis Avenue Bridge. "I was crossing the bridge back into Manhattan," Rodgers recalled, "and Frank was coming over into the Bronx."

He remembered Shorter nodding to him and saying, "Nice going, Bill," as the men symbolically passed each other running in opposite directions. Rodgers would win that day and for the next three years in a row.

Jelena Prokopcuka starts this day trying to become the first woman since Grete Waitz to win three straight titles. Prokopcuka would seem an unlikely repeat champion considering her frail beginnings in the sport and lack of confidence at her first New York City Marathon in 2004.

But Prokopcuka has a ferocity lurking beneath her porcelain exterior. She loves to win. And if she cannot win, she still loves to compete. This mile is where Prokopcuka will find a personal victory today.

She did hit The Wall here in 2004. Knowing that she would be going against a speedier Paula Radcliffe, Prokopcuka nearly conceded victory by hanging in the back of the lead pack. Then, after Mile 20, she withered in the heat and finished fifth. She would learn from the experience.

When Prokopcuka returned to New York in 2005—fresh off her first career marathon victory in Osaka, where she set a Latvian record (2:22:56) that is still her personal best—she got a boost when Radcliffe was not in the race. This time, running a slower pace through 20 miles, Prokopcuka still felt fresh in the Bronx. But after she headed into Harlem off the Madison Avenue Bridge, she suddenly grabbed her side in pain.

In their kitchen in Jurmala before this Marathon, Prokopcuka and her husband re-created the rest of the 2005 race that changed their lives. They completed each other's sentences.

Jelena: "When I turned downhill, maybe this downhill was too hard for me. I had this liver pain. It was . . ."

Aleks: "A very difficult moment. I was so upset."

Jelena: "It was a very difficult moment because, thirty seconds before, I felt so good feelings. I was so strong and then—irk!—I felt my liver spasm."

Aleks: "She started to drop off a little bit."

Jelena continued in breathless English. Susan Chepkemei, of Kenya, who had lost to Radcliffe the year before by three hundredths of a second, was running a few blocks ahead of her with Ethiopian great Derartu Tulu.

"After two or three minutes, my liver recovered, but they were eighteen seconds in front of me. It was difficult to catch them. I wasn't disappointed, because I understood that in front of me would be a hill and I would have a chance to catch them."

Running hills is Jelena's strength.

"When I saw Chepkemei drop off, I understand I could be third. And then when I saw Derartu she was dropping off, I understand that maybe I could catch her, too. And when I caught her, I was feeling good."

Chepkemei had expended her energy too soon around the twenty-third mile. "She started to run very fast," Jelena said. "It's a very difficult moment for the body. Your milk concentration . . ."

"It increases," Aleks said of the lactic-acid buildup.

"It's like a poisoning," Jelena said. She added that she realized it was time for her to take the lead.

"Because it's so famous a run," she says. "I felt my legs were tough, my body was tired. It was warm. But in the last mile, I realized I could win. I wanted to go."

She kept pushing until the finish line appeared magically before her. "Then I saw the last 400 meters, when I could see this blue ribbon in front of me, with the golden, yellow, red leaves—this picture all time before my eyes. It was like a dream. You understand that you are going to . . ."

"Touch a dream," Aleks said.

"It's a really, really unforgettable feeling," Jelena concluded. "Because I cannot imagine it, that I could win the New York City Marathon."

When her body recovered a couple of weeks later and she returned to running in Jurmala, people stopped her on the streets. She was approached for interviews, for sponsorships in Riga. She still has her contract with the local BMW dealer, who, in exchange for an autographed outfit that she wore on race day (it was not the actual one, but one of the many interchangeable ones her sponsor Nike had given her), agreed to lease her and Aleks a sports utility vehicle.

By the time Prokopcuka returned to New York in 2006, she was stronger mentally and physically. Prerace attention focused on Deena Kastor, who set the American marathon record while winning the 2006 London Marathon. But Prokopcuka charged into the spotlight once the race started. She broke from the pack twice in the first half of the race. By the time she got to the Bronx, she was running alone and never had any competition, much to the relief of her anxious parents watching live in Latvia. She won in 2:25:05.

Prokopcuka became a Latvian superstar. She met U.S. President George W. Bush and Latvian President Vaira Vike-Freiberga during the NATO Summit in Riga following the 2006 race. She earned a presidential medal and went to Vike-Freiberga's house. She won her second Latvian Sports Person of the Year award. She says she helped put Latvia on the map, letting people see the face of a country proud of its seas and forests, a country striving to become recognized economically, too, within the European Union.

For all of her fame, however, Prokopcuka has not lost touch with her homespun side. The laurel wreath from her first New York City victory lies on the bottom shelf of her trophy case, the leaves now dried. "Sometimes," she confided with a smile, "I take a leaf for the soap."

A few seconds later, her creative mix-up of English vowels makes sense. "Soup!"

Restaurants in Jurmala serve no fewer than five soups, from borscht to mushroom barley to tomato bisque. Nothing like the sweet taste of victory to make the broth more savory. Today, Prokopcuka knows early she will likely not add to her stock of spices.

She has long legs, like Radcliffe, but not the same, elongated stride. Prokopcuka has one of the most fluid, textbook strides in the women's marathon; it is short and efficient, complementing her perfectly upright carriage. She does not grimace in agony or clench her fists or sit on a competitor's heels. Instead, Prokopcuka seems to be out for a pleasant jog on a Baltic Sea beach just down the block from her house.

Look closely, though, and her stride today will reveal the slightest of hitches. She is favoring her sore left hip. Prokopcuka is nearly a half mile behind the lead pair of women. She realizes that she will neither win nor collect a half-million dollars from the World Marathon Majors.

Why—and how—does a professional athlete, out of the running for the only two real prizes, keep running? She finds someone to pass.

It is a game even a recreational runner will play to make a run matter or come more quickly to its end.

Prokopcuka, Catherine Ndereba and Lidiya Grigoryeva are approaching the orange carpet on the Willis Avenue Bridge. Ndereba made a tactical error five miles earlier on the Queensboro Bridge, when she took off the turtleneck underneath her singlet and lost 12 seconds in the awkward process.

By mile marker 17 on First Avenue, Ndereba uses the downhill slope and crowd excitement to run the fastest split-time of any woman this race: 5:14. But the energy expenditure will cost her. Already Ndereba comes into this race with a compromised physical condition, having won the World Championships in Osaka under oppressively hot and humid conditions just eleven weeks before.

At 35, she is known as Catherine the Great for finishing no worse than third in sixteen of her seventeen marathon starts. She has never won New York, but she has won Boston four times. Plus, she earned a silver at the Athens Olympics and a gold at the 2003 and 2007 World Championships (when Radcliffe did not participate). Today, though, Ndereba's famed durability fades. Prokopcuka surges past her across the Willis Avenue Bridge. One down.

Less than a mile later, just before Prokopcuka approaches the Madison Avenue Bridge going into Manhattan, she picks off Grigoryeva. When Prokopcuka enters Harlem, she knows she is running by herself and for herself. She thinks of her father-in-law, Sergei, who died in July of a heart attack. Before the race, she dedicated her marathon to him. She may not be able to deliver victory, but she intends to give him her best today.

21

BREATHING NEW LIFE

Mile 21, Fifth Avenue, Harlem

Donald Arthur crosses back into Harlem, six hours and twenty-one miles already behind him today. Arthur still has eighty minutes left to walk in his tenth New York City Marathon with the heart of Fitzgerald Gittens pumping inside him.

On August 2, 1996, Gittens, 25, died in a spray of gunfire in the Bronx. He had been headed to his sister's house for dinner when a bullet struck him as he sat in the passenger seat of a friend's car. Gittens's family donated five of his organs that night, sustaining five lives.

At the time of the homicide, Donald Arthur was at home, waiting. It was one week after his fifty-third birthday, and he had been on a heart transplant list for well over a year, since November 1995. He had cardiomyopathy, a disease that causes the heart's walls to weaken and become inflamed, and he was told he would die inside a year without a new heart. Arthur's doctors wasted no time. Four hours after Gittens was gunned down, Arthur was in surgery.

Two months later, in an effort to strengthen his new heart, Arthur started walking. A friend who had also had a heart transplant steered Arthur to the Achilles Track Club, which met regularly for training sessions in Central Park.

"I got there, and I was confronted with people who were blind and had all kinds of situations. I thought, 'What the hell am I doing here? I don't have their problems," Arthur recalled. "I figured I'll go out with them and see what it's like."

He was wearing his work clothes that day. When he started walking with the team members, he saw people mentally and physically challenged, as well as wounded veterans.

"Just that one time I realized that's where I belonged," Arthur said. "Listening to what they had gone through, their resilience and fortitude, they were bouncing back from situations unimaginable, people with one leg and no legs. Just seeing all of this, I realized my pride was my Achilles heel."

He became a racewalker, and in November 1997, at the suggestion of Achilles' founder Dick Traum, he completed his first marathon in New York. "I thought about my donor—I thought that I could fulfill his dream," Arthur said. "At least, that was my driving force, that this would be fulfilling a dream if he had never done one."

Soon after, Arthur wrote a letter to Gittens's mother, Margaret Grady, and his brother, Mack Andrews. "How do you say thank you to someone that saved your life?" Arthur recalled. "There aren't enough words to say it. I remember trying to write the letters. The only thing that filled up the pages was tears."

In 1999, he convinced Andrews to walk the Marathon with him. When they crossed the Verrazano-Narrows Bridge, Arthur took Andrews's hand and slid it under his jersey, telling him: "Feel my heart. Your brother is here with us."

When the pair crossed the finish line in 6 hours, 57 minutes and 21 seconds, Margaret Grady was there. She put medals around both of their necks, the three of them sobbing.

"It never got any better than that," Arthur said.

From there, he started his goal to racewalk a marathon in all fifty states while raising awareness for organ donors. But while his heart was healthy, he had other medical setbacks. In 2003, Arthur was diagnosed with prostate cancer; he continued walking during the radiation treatments that eradicated the cancer.

On Marathon Sunday he is still cancer free, and he already looks ahead to his next marathon. After New York, Arthur will complete the Las Vegas Marathon in December, bringing his 2007 tally to eleven. At 63, he has walked twenty-five marathons in fifteen states. While he has had to stop racewalking because of soreness in his hips, he still walks marathons at a 17-minute per mile pace.

"I don't like to stay on the sidelines," Arthur said with a laugh.

When not training or participating in marathons, he gives speeches urging people to be organ donors. He is buoyed by his new marriage; he remarried two years ago after meeting his wife, Muriel, on the Internet. Arthur may be slowing down, but he will not stop walking.

"I have nothing to prove to anyone," Arthur added. "When I go out there, it's going out to have fun. Being in Central Park in spring and fall, the runners are out there running their backsides off, wondering what's their time, what's their pulse rate. I'm out there seeing new flowers, seeing the leaves starting to change and seeing the beauty of that."

Arthur heard the news about Ryan Shay's fatal heart attack the day before the Marathon. He did not wonder about his own heart, the heart of Fitzgerald Gittens, because his yearly exam was clean.

"Whether it's a heart issue or anything, when an athlete dies, especially those in the same field, it causes you to step back," Arthur said. "You look at life and not take it for granted.

"It comes as a shock, the one thing I deal with and understand,

that death is a part of life, it happens to every living organism. The question I present is, 'Will our death be final?'"

It does not have to be, as Fitzgerald Gittens reminds him today and every day.

W elcome to Harlem! This is how we do it!" shouts the DJ from the stage at the intersection of Fifth Avenue and 135th Street, greeting runners as they come off the Madison Avenue Bridge at Mile Marker 21.

The Marathon course runs along the edge of central Harlem, two avenues away from where Malcom X used to preach on street corners and an enterprising young lawyer named Percy Sutton represented him in the early 1960s. Sutton would become the Manhattan borough president, leading the city through turbulent times from 1966 to 1977.

Sutton already had a daring résumé; he had been a stunt pilot and he flew with the Tuskegee Airmen in World War II. His sense of adventure began at age 12 when he left his home in San Antonio, Texas, by stowing away on a passenger train bound for New York City. His parents made him return to Texas, but Sutton determined then that he would get back to New York—and stay—later in life.

Sutton's intrepid spirit served him well when trying to establish the five-borough marathon. The idea came out of discussions that George Spitz, a runner and city auditor who served on the board of the New York Road Runners club, had with Ted Corbitt. Corbitt, a quiet but passionate proponent of long-distance running, was a 1952 U.S. Olympian in the marathon, and the first president of the club in 1958. Spitz took Corbitt's original proposal of an interborough team competition and turned it into a bicentennial celebration that would close the streets of New York in 1976.

Sutton immediately embraced it. "I wouldn't call it courage," Sutton said. "I had the power at that time. I knew it would be a good idea for the city. It brought vitality. It brought new experiences."

Lebow immediately opposed the idea. Closing Central Park for the four-lap marathon and securing police cooperation had been hard enough, Lebow thought. And he would need $20,000. Sutton promised to procure both money and official support.

When Sutton approached Mayor Abraham D. Beame one day at City Hall in late 1975, the city was still reeling from its fiscal crisis, and Beame indicated he didn't have a dime to spare, let alone $20,000. A couple of days later, Sutton bumped into the real estate magnate Lewis Rudin in the rotunda at City Hall. Rudin had founded the Association for a Better New York in 1971 and had already saved the city once. He had galvanized New York City's top executives to prepay their companies' Manhattan property taxes in 1975, contributing $600 million to the city's shrunken coffers and rescuing New York from potential bankruptcy.

"I have an idea," Sutton said to Rudin, explaining the concept and asking for the money. "Wonderful," Lew replied. "Let's go for it. Let me talk to Jack."

His younger brother, Jack, recalled not giving it a second thought, and they decided to contribute $25,000. Why? "Because it would be good for the city," Jack said, repeating the family motto.

But their interest was personal, too. The Rudins' father, Samuel, had recently passed away; he had been a running enthusiast, a member of the Pastime Athletic Club that met at Macomb's Dam Park in the Bronx where he lived. Jack Rudin recalled his father being a great walker in his later years and a four-wall handball player for the club. The brothers thought sponsoring such a grand athletic event as a marathon would be a fitting monument to Samuel Rudin.

Lew and Jack did more than just contribute money. Lew had influence with company executives and worked with Lebow to get the financial backing of Charlie McCabe, then a vice president of Manufacturers Hanover Trust Company. Meanwhile, Sutton pushed the Marathon idea through the city's agencies, mostly ensuring that the police and fire departments would lend their cooperation.

Yet, despite this momentum, publicity was scarce leading up to the debut of the five-borough marathon.

"We thought maybe we'd get several hundred runners," Jack said. "Nobody thought this would take off. We had some nerve."

Some nerve turned into an economic windfall for the city.

Mayor Michael Bloomberg's office estimated the economic impact for the 2006 Marathon to be $220 million, with the favorable exchange rate for the 20,000 foreigners in 2007 yet to be calculated.

The Netherlands-based financial company, ING, signed a multi-year deal in 2003 to be the title sponsor of the race, while the Rudin family remains a primary sponsor. Lew, a philanthropist beloved throughout the city, died in 2001 of cancer, ten days after the September 11 terrorist attacks. Jack, crediting his brother's "gung ho" spirit for the Marathon, carries it on.

Everyone involved in the race has a personal connection, it seems, and even the most influential leaders like Jack Rudin and Percy Sutton felt drawn to contribute in small, more personal ways.

Rudin, 75, recalled arriving at Fort Wadsworth for the start in 1976 and being flooded with memories. He had been stationed there with the U.S. Army in 1943 for three months before he left for Europe, where he served as a staff sergeant in charge of mortars and machine guns in France, Germany and Czechoslovakia. On the grounds of the fort for the first five-borough marathon, Rudin spotted a colonel, explained his own military background and asked if the colonel could arrange for the Army band to play at the start. Rudin also requested that two cannons be wheeled in on a truck, to signal the beginning of the race with far more of a flourish than a starter's pistol. That tradition has endured.

One year, when funds were too low to support the Army band, Rudin made a phone call to a friend in Washington, D.C., a fellow City College of New York alumnus: Colin Powell. He happened to be chairman of the U.S. Joint Chiefs of Staff at the time, and Powell made sure the band played on.

Rudin also recalled how his brother, Lew, went to Tiffany's in 1976 to have a sterling silver winner's trophy (a tray) designed. The tray varies in size for the top three finishers; a course map, complete with the runners' path from Fort Wadsworth to Tavern on the Green, is engraved in a dotted wavy line. These trays have made their way into homes around the world. Bearing a few fingerprints, the 2005 and 2006 women's trophies sit on Jelena Prokopcuka's crowded bookshelf in Latvia. The 2004 men's trophy rests on Hendrick Ramaala's coffee table in South Africa next to which his son, Alex, has spread his Disney books and DVDs.

Closer to home, Sutton said he is proud of his own contributions to the city, even if he never realized his dream of becoming mayor. Two months after the 2007 Marathon, the stretch of course between the Mile 21 and Mile 22 markers, all on Fifth Avenue, will be renamed Honorable Percy E. Sutton Way.

Sutton had founded the Inner City Broadcasting Corporation which, before going on to run the Apollo Theater, bought the first black-owned radio station in New York City, WLIB in Harlem. During the first few years of the five-borough marathon, Sutton said he helped choose uplifting songs for the station to broadcast live, with outdoor speakers positioned along Fifth Avenue.

Sutton, now 87, cannot recall what songs he requested to be played, only that they were, as he said with a chuckle, "audacious."

Today, an R&B singer named Orikl, performs at 126th Street and Fifth Avenue, followed by the Washington Irving High School drum line. Children have written encouragement in multicolored chalk on the street, but thousands of pounding feet will eventually smudge the words so that only "Go!" is recognizable.

22

VICTORY ONE

Marcus Garvey Park to 103rd Street and Fifth Avenue

Two men grip the ends of the Ethiopian flag and tear down the sidewalk along Fifth Avenue in a blur of green, yellow and red, chasing Ethiopia's Gete Wami, who is chasing Great Britain's Paula Radcliffe. As she has been for most of the race, Radcliffe is still a step ahead of Wami as they turn into Marcus Garvey Park, just approaching the marker for Mile 22. Wami's impromptu fan club of two nimbly dodges light poles and fire hydrants without injuring important body parts, all while shaking the flag tautly in their hands.

Ethiopia is the oldest independent country in Africa never to have been colonized, and its tricolor flag has become recognized as the colors of the continent. Marcus Garvey, who argued that those of African ancestry could return to redeem Africa, had lived in Harlem and would have been proud of the display.

During the years of World War I, Garvey moved to New York from Jamaica, preaching from street corners the radical ideas of racial separatism and self-reliance. He advocated the liberation of Africa from colonial rule and supported the notion that a black king would lead Africa. In 1930, Haile Selassie was crowned Emperor of Ethiopia.

When Wami arrives on the edge of Marcus Garvey Park today at 122nd Street and Fifth Avenue, she is proud to represent Ethiopia, but she cannot allow herself to be distracted by acknowledging her two fans. She is running a 5-minute, 34-second mile. The men, their chests heaving, give up the trail halfway around the park.

Will Wami be able to sustain her quest?

Grete Waitz, in the red convertible pace car, wants to know. When her car pulls even to the press truck, Waitz gives a wave and shouts, "Who do you think?"

Radcliffe is the answer, with a caveat: Wami is still looking strong.

What does the nine-time New York City Marathon champion think?

"Paula," Waitz says with a simple smile and a nod. She knows something about this game. She and Radcliffe still share the same physiotherapist, Gerard Hartmann, in Ireland. They share the same background running races on the track, and many of the same credentials.

Waitz broke her own world record twice in New York but was never able to match this success in the Olympics. In the inaugural women's Olympic marathon in 1984, she finished second, 400 meters behind Joan Benoit, who became the beloved American superstar. Twenty years later at the Athens Olympics, Radcliffe would drop out of the marathon in agony—at Mile 22. She has never lost a marathon she has finished.

Like Waitz, Radcliffe has had her own string of dominance in New York. Coming into today, she has won four straight races here, starting with two victories in the Fifth Avenue Mile, one in the 2001 Mini 10K and another in the 2004 Marathon. The only race Radcliffe lost in this city was her first Fifth Avenue Mile, in 1995. She confessed that perhaps she and her future husband, Gary Lough, should not have been so busy being tourists beforehand, going to the top of the Empire State Building and walking around the city. Radcliffe lost by only six-hundredths of a second.

Now Radcliffe and Wami round the corner of the park, turning back onto Fifth Avenue for the long uphill stretch before they enter Central Park. Neither is ready to make any move yet, each knowing that the opportunity will likely not appear for another three miles. They proceed at a bit slower pace (5:34), trying to ignore the heaviness that is starting to settle into their legs. At 1468 Fifth Avenue, between 118th and 117th streets, Radcliffe and Wami pass a senior housing facility. No one has come outside yet to cheer the runners, because it is still early in the race day here. But the name above the door to the apartment building speaks louder than any fan could: Victory One.

Here, in a nondescript mile without many fans, beginning a tortuous climb where the body flashes warning signs of shutdown, each runner must find his or her inner strength. The Marathon at this point becomes not the fervent communal cause that Garvey championed, nor a grand parade marching through Brooklyn nor a swarm moving up Manhattan's First Avenue. Here is where victory truly hinges on the power of one.

The lead pack of the men's professional race has dwindled from the dozen who started the First Avenue stretch in Manhattan, to five in the Bronx—Rodgers Rop, James Kwambai, Martin Lel, Abderrahim Goumri and Hendrick Ramaala. After a flurry of activity in the twenty-second mile, the pack will soon be three.

Rop, the 2002 champion, should have been in prime position.

But the combination of Hendrick Ramaala's surging on First Avenue and Rop's pacing of Haile Gebrselassie to the world record (through 18.6 miles) five weeks earlier in Berlin has left him nothing in reserve. He drops off in this mile.

James Kwambai suffered from a bout of malaria as he was leaving Kenya for the Berlin Marathon at the end of September. He missed that race and in this one begins to slow with each step, falling five seconds and then eleven seconds behind a lead pack that has shed its excess weight and is now only three—Ramaala, Lel and Goumri.

Suddenly, Lel and Goumri make it a party of two, breaking aggressively from Ramaala as they turn around the square-shaped Marcus Garvey Park and start to head back up Fifth Avenue. The picture is eerily familiar, even if Goumri has only recently become part of such a scene.

Goumri, a compact 5 foot 6, 124 pounds, began his running career in the mid-nineties competing on the track and in cross-country competitions; he had never won a major international race. He did run a marathon once, on a whim, but that was back in 1997, when he won Norway's Midnight Sun Marathon in 2 hours, 30 minutes—a pedestrian time even for an elite woman. Still, Goumri was asked after that victory if he intended to make the marathon his specialty.

"No," he replied, then 21 years old. "I am from Morocco. I am a 1,500-meter and 5,000-meter runner."

At that time, Morocco already had a legendary middle-distance runner in the making—Hicham El-Guerrouj—who would go on to win four straight world championship gold medals in the 1,500 meters and gold medals in both the 1,500 and 5,000 meters at the 2004 Athens Olympics.

Goumri eventually realized that with El-Guerrouj ahead of him and middle distance events loaded in talent with other African runners, he had best find another race. In 2006 he hired his training partner, the 2000 New York City Marathon champion from Morocco, Abdelkhader el-Mouaziz, to coach him in the marathon. The two lived at the high-altitude training center in Ifrane, Morocco, and trained on rough trails in the Atlas Mountains, 8,800 feet above sea level.

Goumri's results were immediate in his new distance running. Not counting the blip on his résumé in Norway, Goumri made a splash in his official big-city marathon debut at London in April 2007. There, he and Lel ran in a tight pack of six runners, including Ramaala, with less than three miles to go. The pack became four, and in the final 200 meters, Lel surged in front. Goumri was the only one to follow. Lel shrugged off his competitor's move and stormed to the tape, beating Goumri by a three-second margin, in 2:07:41.

Goumri entered one more marathon before New York—the World Championships in Osaka. He was feeling good until he was besieged by cramps past the halfway mark and dropped out of the race. He was already thinking he needed to save himself for New York.

Today, as Lel and Goumri grab their water bottles on the edge of Harlem, Ramaala uses their deceleration to catch the pair. When they turn onto the incline of Fifth Avenue in the twenty-third mile, Ramaala again slips in behind them as the trio passes Central Park's Conservatory Garden at 105th Street.

Ramaala's T-shirt is untucked and his right elbow looks as if it is duct-taped to his side. Both running styles are his trademark. Ramaala drops his arms when tired, but his right arm droops lower. His wife, Rodica, thinks he does this to compensate for one leg being longer than the other. Ramaala says his orthotics specially made of phone books are supposed to correct that. He is used to running this way and far too tired to care now. Ramaala is approaching Mile Marker 23, at 103rd Street. His energy is ebbing, but he tells himself he is not out of the race yet.

Harrie is, by this point, definitely out of it. On the agonizing climb up Fifth Avenue, he realizes he has nothing left. Regardless of the classes he took, the miles he logged, the gels he ingested, the Gatorade and water he dutifully drank, Harrie hits The Wall, because he has never gone this far on his feet in his life.

"Just no energy and a lack of willpower," he will describe the problem later, referring to sensations that under rational circumstances he never lacks. Everything feels just very foggy.

A couple of miles earlier, his lower back started to bother him, which had never happened in any of his long runs before. The bottoms of his feet are aching, and he gets a strain in his neck, on the left side, the opposite side of the scar. He is cold. It's not that he's unhappy; he is just hurting. OK, maybe he is a little unhappy. He can sense his best friend and brother next to him, dragging him onward.

"We are so close. You are so strong. You look so great," Rich says.

"OK," Harrie mumbles, trying to believe his brother, but mostly just trying to plant one foot in front of the other.

Two weeks earlier, Harrie ran the final 10 miles of the Marathon course with his brother, Rich, and forty Fred's Team members. Lynn Bradley, their 30-year-old teammate with a sunny Scottish lilt, paced them both in the final miles. She told the brothers to sprint up Fifth Avenue into Central Park to make themselves so tired that they would replicate the conditions of the Marathon. Harrie was beaming after that October training run; he had run the final three miles at a 6:30 pace.

He feels nothing like that day and cannot even summon its memory now. Harrie is trudging on at an 11-minute pace and just wants to get to Central Park. There, at least he knows he will finish.

The Fifth Avenue incline is not the steepest, but it is the most brutal hill on the course because of its timing; runners hit this subtle incline just when they are suffering the most. With each passing light pole, the Fifth Avenue stretch of the course seems to be extending, like some devilish optical illusion.

In a perverse way, Pam Rickard loves this hill, just as she has enjoyed conquering all of them today. They give her a chance to pass people. Having trained on the rolling hills beneath the Blue Ridge Mountains of Virginia, Pam has no problem climbing today.

To help speed her along, her husband, Tom, is waiting to encourage her at their second designated meeting spot of the race. At the first, 100th Street and First Avenue, Tom's booming cry of "Pam!" ricocheted off the buildings, and everybody from the Bronx to Queens could probably hear him. He is a part-time announcer at local road races and triathlons in Roanoke, but today his deep, resonant voice speaks to Pam alone.

"It is well with my soul, baby!" she shouts back on 100th Street.

By the time Tom sees her again on Fifth Avenue, he notices a change in her face. Pam is not in pain, but she is grimly determined. It is not enough for her just to finish; she must finish purposefully.

Even before she arrived in New York, Pam felt reborn as a runner. After particularly long workouts, she would experience a runner's high, a phenomenon that German researchers in early 2008 would prove exists. Pam felt pure joy from running, but mostly, she was relieved simply to be able to feel again. With no alcohol in her system, she could again sense every knee pain, the burn from every hill, the sting of every sunburn.

"It's just this overall feeling of being clean is so amazing," she said. "Alcohol, it's a poison to my body."

Free of such poison, she can run now without nausea as her constant companion, without stopping to unload her lunch. She can run without excuses and gauge the importance of every mile completed. "Living in truth" has helped her become a better athlete.

Humility does not come naturally to her. She admitted to what she called "the defects in my character," the arrogance and the fear that led her to disappear into herself and abandon her family. She would check herself regularly, maintaining her sobriety with the same discipline she needed to run this marathon.

There have been small victories along the way as her children attempted to move on as well. Rachel decided to join the cross-country team in her freshman year of high school. When she could get a ride to practice, Pam occasionally helped out as a volunteer coach, and Rachel no longer pretended not to know her.

"Our sport is your sport's punishment," read the back of Rachel's cross-country team shirt in the fall of 2007. She was proud to wear it. She was surprisingly happy running, and Pam was silently thrilled she chose it on her own.

Sophie, a clever and affectionate four-year-old, retained her rambunctious spirit.

The biggest change occurred in Abby, who never felt close to her mother until now. She arrived at Virginia Tech as a freshman in September, to a place that, itself, was trying to heal after the horrific shooting spree of the previous spring. Abby, who earned a significant academic scholarship to attend the school, came to college having recently repaired her fractured relationships with her mother and her boyfriend of three years. She said she decided to try "this whole God thing," and although she was a skeptic at first, she gradually began to gain a sense of calm and clarity that helped her forgive her mother.

Her relationship grew even stonger with her boyfriend. And she made one bold decision: to stop drinking.

There have been some difficult days still for Pam, and the running has helped calm her restlessness. The family's finances have been tight on Tom's teacher salary alone. Pam volunteered as a fundraiser for the county's new library and still had to rely on rides to get her out of the house. But while running once distanced her from her family, it has since helped her feel connected to them again.

Abby used to resent her mother's running. "Now, I feel like she runs for the love of running," Abby said. "And I see the sheer joy and closeness to God it brings her, and I truly could not be happier for her."

In her newly conscious state of sobriety, Pam seems to notice signs in everyday life, both spiritual and mundane. Here at Mile 22—farther than Pam has run in a single day over the past eight years—she pushes past her weariness, summoning the motivation that will bring her home. Her path has already been filled with powerful signposts telling her she will finish, like the one she stumbled upon six weeks earlier.

The sun was beaming beneath the blanket of a cerulean sky as a few white jet plumes interrupted the perfection. It was early fall in southern Virginia, and Pam was running past broken-down tractors, the Blue Ridge Mountains spread richly around her. She ran by fields of corn waiting to be harvested and saw only one car on the double-lane county road. Dogs barked shrilly in the distance. She charged uphill past trees, their bottom branches heavy at the base with cocoons. Pam did not notice them; she had spent enough time inside one.

Out on the solitary roads, with her iPod playing Christian rock, and her feet gliding over the asphalt, Pam knew she was on the right path. Except that on this day, in the middle of a 10-mile solo run on roads near her house she had crossed for more than a decade, Pam really needed a water station.

She had neglected to bring any water with her, thinking she would be fine without it. She could still be stubborn that way, and because of her short-sightedness she was getting dehydrated. As Pam approached her 5-mile turnaround spot, she decided to take a shortcut through the fields of the Gogginsville United Methodist Church.

As she rounded the corner into the empty fields, she looked to her left and suddenly spotted three wooden crosses that she had never seen before. She looked closer. And there, to the side of the crosses, was a water pump, with a 3-foot hose attached. It was no mirage.

Overcome with delight and gratitude, she stopped, pumped and drank eagerly of the coldest, clearest and sweetest liquid she could remember. As the water cascaded down her throat, it cleansed her soul in a most private epiphany.

23

LUNGS OF NEW YORK

Mile 23, Fifth Avenue to Central Park

Luxurious apartment buildings from the 1920s, museums and mansions line the east side of Fifth Avenue as the runners climb their way up a corridor of money and memory. On the opposite side of the street, stately elm trees, as well as the orange Marathon route banners hanging from light poles become markers on Mile 23. Runners look to them to prove to their addled brains that they are making progress, even if their legs seem stuck in poured cement.

Somewhere in Central Park, the finish line beckons like a distant promise.

Just before 97th Street, Hendrick Ramaala concedes defeat. His 35-year-old legs, exhausted from his surges today, can no longer keep pace with Abderrahim Goumri and Martin Lel, who are still running as smoothly as they did at the opening miles of the race. They hide their leg pain well at least.

Goumri's biggest problem now is his mind. He knows Lel has the strongest finishing kick in the marathon business. *Do I go now? Or save my move for later?* Goumri wonders.

Each time Goumri tries a mini surge on Fifth Avenue, Lel covers it. Goumri gambles and opts to save his bigger move for later, while Lel salivates and gains confidence with every step they share.

Ramaala will watch their backs grow smaller as they gain a lead of one block, two blocks, three blocks and then 30 seconds as they turn right into Central Park at 90th Street. Ramaala cannot afford to slow down; his race is far from over. Ramaala is striving toward a more personal goal—today he can still capture a spot on the South African Olympic team if he runs below 2 hours and 12 minutes. If he were to push harder right now to stay with Lel and Goumri, he might fall farther in the final miles, maybe to fourth or fifth place, and not qualify.

South Africa has not won an Olympic marathon medal since Josia Thugwane captured gold at the 1996 Atlanta Summer Games, the first year South Africa returned to international competition after the end of apartheid. The country was delirious over his medal.

"Maybe it is because we have many gold mines that gold is worshipped," Ramaala surmised. "Silver? What's silver? What's bronze?

"They thought he would win lots of medals," he added, shaking his head. Thugwane instead became caught in the glare of fame and was never able to build off his amazing race.

Pride, the fool's gold of competition, was why Ramaala ran the entire world championship marathon in Osaka, Japan, in sweltering heat the previous August. He had dropped out of two previous world championships and endured the stinging media criticism. Who were others to say that Ramaala did not love his country?

Even though he endangered his body in Osaka by running while dehydrated, he did not want to be remembered as a quitter. Instead, Ramaala finished twenty-seventh, running a painful 2:26, and was one of the few top professionals to finish the race. Over the grueling 26.2 miles, he kept telling himself it would be good preparation for similar conditions in Beijing—that if he survived this, he would be able to win an Olympic medal.

Survival came with a price though. For nearly five weeks afterward, Ramaala struggled to recover. His upper body felt tight, as if the oppressive heat and humidity were still lodged in his chest and shoulders.

Ramaala did not regret his decision to finish, because the international competitions are what ultimately motivate him. "For me, that's how I started," he said. "I still get excited going to world championships. I love to see a medal. If I win a medal for this country, I would be very happy.

"It has," Ramaala added, "nothing to do with money."

The conflict between money and purity always seems to simmer near the surface of this sport. Road running is a fickle business. Only the top elite marathoners—competing usually in just two 26.2-mile races per year and a handful of road races at shorter distances—can earn close to $2 million a year in prize money, appearance fees and endorsements. But stumble through a winless marathon season and the financial consequences are inevitable.

Nike did not renew Ramaala's contract after he failed to follow up his 2004 New York City victory; he then signed with Adidas. Ramaala earned close to six figures from the New York Road Runners to appear in today's race; it was not the top appearance fee, but one that took into account his past success in New York.

Paula Radcliffe, the world record holder and the athlete who today draws a live BBC television audience back in the UK, earned more than three times that in appearance fees today. In addition to public prize money and bonuses for running under a certain time (such as 2:21, 2:22), each athlete's agent negotiates separate time bonuses (such as if the athlete is first after certain points on the course) as part of the overall package. Marathon organizers and agents do not publicly disclose these packages in order to retain bargaining power, but they have long been a source of gossip and contention in the industry.

Although Radcliffe's success affords her and her husband a comfortable lifestyle in tax-free Monaco, when her feet hit the New York pavement and her head starts nodding, it is business as usual for her. She is focused solely on that finish line. Her unequivocal desire to win is so fierce that perhaps only her husband can match it.

Gary Lough is in a frantic state. His wife has made what seemed to be her first major move away from Gete Wami on Fifth Avenue, just before the pair entered the park. With crowds screaming beside her, Radcliffe surged 10 meters ahead and then 20 meters ahead—her biggest lead of the race.

Just then, WNBC, the local television affiliate carrying the race live, cut to commercial. Lough, watching on a few different screens in a VIP room at Tavern on the Green, is outraged and in agony. He presses speed dial on his cell phone to call someone, anyone watching the live feed on the BBC. He reaches his parents, Dale and Sally, in Ballygally, Northern Ireland.

"She's got a break, got a gap!" Sally informs her son.

But from the background, Lough can hear his dad shout, "No she hasn't, no she hasn't!"

Lough is beside himself with the conflicting reports. Why didn't he just call his brother? Why didn't the feed stay live in the VIP room?

Mostly, he is questioning his wife for not breaking away from Wami. Lough is still remembered for his spat, caught on camera at the 2001 World Track and Field Championships in Edmonton. In the stadium tunnel, he yelled at his devastated wife minutes after she finished fourth in the 10,000 meters—eight hundredths of a second behind Wami. He wondered then why she hadn't made a move earlier, according to their prerace plan. Radcliffe pushed him away.

Six years later in their coaching and domestic relationship, Lough now tries to calm himself down as he desperately waits for the Marathon coverage to return. "I'm trying to put myself in her position," he will recall. "If she knew she had gotten a break, she would have done something. She was thinking—leave it for later."

This is true. Radcliffe, in fact, has no idea how large her lead is on Wami, since she has not seen her all day behind her. And her legs are starting to stiffen, slowing her pace only so slightly. The conditions are not ideal for a break.

As soon as Radcliffe makes the right turn into the park, the fans are gathered so intimately, they seem to be screaming into her ears.

"The crowd noise was so loud, I didn't realize I had broken away," Radcliffe will say. "If I knew, I probably would have gone."

Enthusiastic, flag-waving, cowbell-ringing fans stacked along both sides of Central Park's two-lane East Drive add another meaning to the popular description of the city's 843-acre oasis—the lungs of New York.

Nowhere in the city is oxygen more plentiful, thanks to the 26,000 trees, from elms to Norway maples and 150-year-old willow oaks. Marathoners seem to breathe easier once they enter the green sanctuary. Maybe this is because they just topped one of the meanest hills on the course. Or maybe, for local runners, it is because they feel as though they are finally in familiar territory.

"Come on—you only have a couple miles left!" a fan shouts to

New Yorker Harrie Bakst. This does not sit very well with Harrie, who, after having already traversed 23 miles through five boroughs, believes he hears a bit of mocking in the cheer.

"Do you want to do this?" he feels like yelling to the warm and relaxed fan, if only he had the energy.

From the southeast corner of East 90th Street and Fifth Avenue, the bells ring at the Church of the Heavenly Rest. Not so fast.

Runners may enjoy a relatively flat quarter-mile once they enter the park, with Frank Lloyd Wright's cylindrical masterpiece, the Guggenheim Museum, looming on their left before they reach the backyard of the sprawling Metropolitan Museum of Art. But after a small uphill, the road will wind painfully downhill out of the park, putting more stress on oozing blisters, throbbing quadriceps and creaking knees.

Before runners realize they still have a haul left, they can at least enjoy the illusion that they are close when they enter Central Park at the Engineers' Gate. One of eighteen original names for entrances to the park, Engineers' Gate is known more informally as runners' gate. On weekday evenings and weekend mornings, virtually every running club, team or class meets here in the clearing beneath the 1.58-mile Jacqueline Kennedy Onassis Reservoir path. The nearly life-size statue of New York City Marathon founder Fred Lebow stands here, checking his watch, timing the masses running past him. (During the week of the Marathon, Lebow's statue is always moved to the finish line at West Drive and 67th Street.)

There are easily more than 5,000 runners in the park on any given autumn weeknight at 7:30 p.m., and the crowds are going both clockwise and counterclockwise—with packs of cyclists whizzing by them at 25 miles an hour.

It is loosely controlled chaos, runners of all body types and abilities training for different distances, from 5Ks to half-marathons to ultramarathons to triathlons. As a middle-aged 7-minute-miler termed it one day: "It's democracy in motion!"

Although Central Park no longer represents the genteel haven Frederick Law Olmsted and his architect partner, Calvert Vaux, had hoped to create with their Greensward Plan of 1858, today's version does capture the spirit of their grand vision. They wanted to provide New Yorkers with a wide-open green space that would enable them to enjoy the aesthetics of landscape art, watch the world go by and engage in exercise.

Olmsted and Vaux's Victorian-era network of grassy fields, dirt trails, lakes, bridges and roads has turned into a vibrant recreational playground. From cricket to volleyball, softball to handball, soccer to tennis, people who don't run have plenty of choices. On weekends and summer weeknights, more sedentary New Yorkers turn the Sheep Meadow on the south end into an urban beach, with stunning views of the affluent apartment buildings lining Central Park West.

The park was not always a metropolitan refuge, however. Rather, during the seventies and eighties, it reflected the city's own unease, becoming a den of crime and violence after dark. The park's reputation hit its nadir thanks to one notorious crime involving a runner.

On the night of April 19, 1989, at around 9 p.m., a female investment banker in her late twenties was jogging in the upper reaches of Central Park when she was raped and beaten, then left for dead near the 102nd Street Transverse. She was in a coma for twelve days.

Amid the nationwide shock and horror over "the Central Park Jogger," the New York Road Runners club immediately worked with city law enforcement officials, the Deparment of Parks and Recreation and the Central Park Conservancy to form its safety patrol. Pairs of runners or street-clothed volunteers took walkie-talkies to survey the trails and roads and reported suspicious activity to the police. By the late nineties, with the further impetus of Mayor Rudy Giuliani's crackdown on crime, the Road Runners' patrol had assisted plainclothes policemen to help make the park safe again.

The Central Park Jogger, herself, was a beneficiary. She recovered and returned, anonymously, to run the New York City Marathon in 1995. Trisha Meili did not publicly reveal her identity until 2003, when she published her memoir, *I Am the Central Park Jogger: A Story of Hope and Possibility*.

As part of her rehabilitation, Meili had joined a chapter of the Achilles Track Club for disabled runners at Gaylord Hospital in Connecticut. She ran a Road Runners' 10-mile race in December 1991 and then she started volunteering at Saturday morning Achilles Track Club runs that met at the Engineers' Gate. Only a few people in the club knew her identity. In 1994, Meili walked the New York City Marathon as a guide for Dick Traum, the founder of Achilles and an above-the-knee amputee who participated in the Marathon wearing a prosthetic; they finished together in just under twelve hours. That race inspired Meili to run the next year.

"I wasn't doing it because I felt like I had to prove something," said Meili, now 47 and chairman of the Achilles Track Club's board. "I was really so happy that I could run."

When Meili entered Central Park for the 1995 Marathon at 102nd Street (the course has since changed), she thought about how close she was to the attack site and felt a surge of energy. She forgot about knee pain and fatigue and felt as if she had reclaimed a part of herself.

"I felt so proud of all the hard work that had gotten me there," Meili said. "In that moment, running those last miles, I knew I would finish it. I felt this tremendous sense of triumph. Here I am. I can do this. In spite of what's happened, I had every right to be there."

The temperature dropped to 33 degrees Fahrenheit during the 1995 race—still an all-time low for the Marathon—as Meili finished in 4 hours, 30 minutes and 1 second.

"Everybody should do it," said Meili, who felt she needed to run the race only once. "Just to have that feeling of all these strangers cheering you on and supporting you—you realize how powerful it is."

The transformative power of running is on full display in Central Park during weekend races and Marathon training sessions, which draw more than 5,000 people for each event. Amid the bustling crowd, one face is always recognizable.

Mary Wittenberg, the Road Runners president and chief executive, can be seen during the forty-some races in Central Park going into an all-out kick to the finish line, her brow furrowed as she blows by people left and right and stops her watch the instant she crosses the line. A minute later, Wittenberg is running back onto the course in the opposite direction to cheer in the next wave, shouting to some by name, others by number.

Wittenberg's second office is Central Park, just across the street from the Road Runners' headquarters on East 89th Street. If the Park is the lungs of the city, then Wittenberg is the bellows of New York's running community.

At 5:30 a.m., just before sunrise, Wittenberg can be found on the bridle path, breathing in the calm, invigorating air. The rising sun throws off the canopy of darkness—not gradually, but in a sudden, fluorescent instant. It is her visual alarm clock for another demanding workday.

Though Wittenberg may start her run with only a few dozen runners around her, by the time she finishes, she is surrounded by hundreds, including many of New York's top executives, lawyers and traders, all getting in a few miles before the day envelops them.

"This is where all the decisions are made at the break of dawn," said Toby Tanser, a coach and former professional runner from Sweden. He often spots Eli Zabar, the gourmet food mogul, in conversation. "It's the think tank of the city."

Welcome to the power breakfast. And as chief executive of a burgeoning organization and the only female race director of the five major international marathons, Wittenberg belongs at the table.

With help from a dedicated core of executives, Wittenberg has grown Road Runners into a formidable brand that has a monopoly on running events in the city and has its sights on growing the brand throughout the world.

Some local runners decry that the Road Runners (which started phasing out the word *club* in its name in 2001) has taken on a corporate identity despite its status as a nonprofit organization. Road Runners reported a projected operating budget of $38 million in 2007, with more than $20 million directed toward the Marathon.

Road Runners has dropped smaller races from the schedule and charges somewhat expensive entry fees (a bit less for members) to run the prime races in the sixty-six-plus annual event calendar in all five city boroughs. That didn't stop membership from expanding by nearly 4,000 runners in 2007, to 45,335.

Members have a local privilege as well: they can gain automatic entry into the Marathon by running nine sanctioned races in the previous year. (In order to gain entry into the 2009 Marathon, members have had to run nine races, plus volunteer at a tenth.) A total of 4,145 Road Runners members were eligible for 2007 through this guaranteed entry.

The 2007 Marathon cost $100 for members and $130 for non-Road Runners members, not including the $20 transportation fee.

Wittenberg argues that not only are these fees appropriate for the overall experience of the Marathon, but revenue from race entry fees throughout the year helps fund programs to educate runners.

"The more money we have, the more we're able to do, the more we're able to support," Wittenberg said.

Her biggest push in the last three years has been on the elite athlete front. In order to bring the sport of running to the mainstream, Wittenberg believes U.S. stars must be marketed like baseball and football players (she thinks big), but first their talent must be developed. For this reason, the Road Runners funds elite training groups all over the country, whether in Boulder, Colorado; suburban Detroit; Minneapolis; or Mammoth Lakes, California.

One Marathon charity is reserved specifically for funding these programs. Runners can pay $2,500 for entry via an elite charity level, the Champions Circle. Today, eighty-five runners will gain entry this way, raising $170,000 for U.S. distance running.

Three Olympic hopefuls, Ryan Hall, Dathan Ritzenhein and Brian Sell, whose training groups the Road Runners aided directly, ran the marathons of their lives Saturday to qualify for the Beijing Games during the U.S. trials in Central Park. The future of American distance running never seemed so promising on November 3. But even as these young stars of the sport were celebrating their achievements, they were also mourning a friend and the flip side of an unforgettable day in Central Park.

24

WHAT PRICE GLORY?

Ryan Shay (1979–2007)

Mile 24 Sunday; Mile 5 Saturday

The stampede rushes south toward the finish line—a life force surging downhill through Central Park, washing over the sorrow of Saturday and flowing past the exact place where Ryan Shay's heart had stopped in a sudden, sickening instant.

Today, that place is between Mile 24 and Mile 25 of the New York City Marathon, on the east side of the road some 200 feet north of the Loeb Boathouse, across from the fire hydrant. In Saturday's Olympic trials, it was a half mile past Mile Marker 5. A 28-year-old elite athlete, a former national marathon champion, was not supposed to die in perfectly cool weather after running 5.5 miles—let alone after any mile, in any weather.

For the professional and recreational marathoners who had listened to the news or perhaps heard the hushed buzz at the New York Marathon Health and Fitness Expo in the Javits Center Saturday afternoon, Shay's death was, of course, shocking. But it was also so rare—no U.S. athlete had ever died trying to qualify for an Olympic team. And it was still so inexplicable that many runners could not relate.

At the technical meeting for the professionals Saturday afternoon, race director Mary Wittenberg made a brief, somber announcement, and then handed the microphone to the elite athlete coordinator, David Monti. Matter-of-factly, he switched to a discussion of minutiae that included water-bottle retrieval and transportation to the start. He reflected the runners' prerace mentality; in order to make it to the starting line the next day, they needed to distance themselves from the improbable tragedy.

Left unspoken were the questions elite athletes would not allow themselves to address until after the race. How far can they push their bodies? Their sport requires them to drive themselves past their physical limits in order to achieve. But will they know when to stop?

"I wonder," Hendrick Ramaala would say walking through sunny Central Park on the Monday after the New York City Marathon, "for sure, you get some sign? There must be some signs before. If there is some breath—uh-huh—and you just run and drop dead? No pain or nothing?

"We're all wondering—it's not just me. If he drops dead and that's it, then we all drop dead and that's it?"

Paramedics recorded that Shay's heart stopped within 15 minutes after he collapsed on November 3, 2007. It took until March 18, 2008, for the New York Medical Examiner's Office to release the results of the autopsy, and even those were inconclusive. Shay died of natural causes after his heart went into an irregular rhythm; his heart was enlarged and showed patchy scars, signs of previous damage. But neither the medical examiner nor genetic specialists could determine when or how the damage occurred.

The damage might have been genetic. Or perhaps it could have been caused by the pneumonia that Shay had when he was 14. It was then that a doctor also discovered he had an enlarged heart. An enlarged heart is not uncommon since some athletes' hearts grow stronger, and thus bigger, because of vigorous exercise. But other enlarged hearts are a result of a genetic condition known as hypertrophic cardiomyopathy, the leading cause of sudden death in young athletes.

Steroids and amphetamines, of course, are also associated with sudden death in athletes. With the sport of track and field tainted recently by revelations of illegal performance-enhancing drug use—most notably Olympic sprinting champion Marion Jones's admission of guilt in October, which would lead to her jail sentence—any remarkable result or tragic turn seems to prompt speculation. Shay's death raised eyebrows in the running community because it was so unfathomable.

(Drug testing occurs at every major track event in the United States, even as some athletes, including Jones, have learned how to cheat the system. In New York, the top three athletes who qualified for the U.S. Olympic marathon team, plus the fourth-place finisher, were tested with a urine sample immediately after the race by the United States Anti-Doping Agency. No athlete would test positive for performance-enhancing drugs.

In Sunday's New York City Marathon, the top three men and top three women, plus two others randomly selected from the top ten finishers, would also be tested for performance-enhancing drugs by a urine test. None of these tests came back positive, either. Blood-testing, which checks for the use of red blood cell–boosting agents such as erythropoietin, was not conducted after the Olympic trials or the New York Marathon.)

Reflecting on Shay's death, the day after his own race, Ramaala would talk of the importance of providing a solid medical explanation, in order to quiet the inevitable speculation about potential drug usage: "If there is no conclusion, people are going to come to their own conclusion, which is sad," Ramaala said.

Four months later, Shay's autopsy would ultimately deflate that speculation, which those closest to him had immediately dismissed: A toxicology screen would show no evidence of performance-enhancing drugs in Shay's body. "He would have quit the sport before using drugs," said Joe Piane, Shay's coach at the University of Notre Dame.

Shay's belief in the purity of sport and his unconditional passion for distance running defined him, as did his nickname, Workhorse.

In life, Shay was a runner for whom the podiums at the big marathons seemed just out of reach. But in dying on the sport's main stage, the U.S. Olympic trials, he attained virtual cult status. Running clubs would hold memorial Ryan Shay 5.5 mile runs across the country, and for three straight nights in Shay's hometown of Central Lake, Michigan, people would walk and run around the high school track as they participated in a candlelight vigil. More than 500 mourners would cram into a small church to attend his funeral. People may not have understood why Shay died, but they understood how he lived to run.

Ryan Shay grew up the third youngest of eight children in a running household, with a father who was a demanding track coach. Joe Shay would admit after the death of his son that he could never again use his favorite slogan:

"Running won't kill you; it will just make you pass out."

Shay seemed to internalize the message but take it a hundred steps farther. "The hardest thing that I learned while coaching Ryan was not telling him what to do, but how to hold him back," Piane said. When he told Shay to run five miles at a certain pace, Shay would ask to run seven miles. "I think he realized he was not the most talented runner on the planet," Piane said, "and so he had to outwork everyone."

Shay did not have the naturally slight build of a distance runner. He was a little more solid at 5-foot-10, 150 pounds. He won eight Michigan state high school championships, and at Notre Dame was a nine-time All-American in track and cross-country. He turned to the marathon after graduation and sparked new hope in American distance running by winning the 2003 U.S. marathon championship in 2:14:29. He also won titles in the half-marathon, the 20 kilometers race and the 15 kilometers race.

But when Shay struggled with injuries after these races, he would only work harder. "If he wasn't feeling well, number one, he would never tell anybody," said Joe Vigil, his postcollegiate coach in the Team USA running program at Mammoth Lakes, California. "He would try to push it more, because he thought he was getting weak.

"I'd chew him out, saying, 'You're doing everything you can. There's only so much the body can take.'"

At one point early in 2006, Shay's body did break down. He was found to have adrenal fatigue syndrome; hormones secreted by the adrenal gland had caused his muscle tissue to weaken. It is often a result of overtraining, and Shay had to cut back for six weeks.

By the time he got to September 2007, Shay knew he was a long shot to make the U.S. Olympic Team. He would likely have to run at least three minutes faster than his personal best, and Shay had not had promising results leading up to the trials. He felt that his body was not recovering as quickly as it once did, and he was losing weight. He complained to his father he had been dizzy, and then Ryan suggested that he not come to New York.

"He told me, 'I don't think I am going to do very well. If it's not there, I am going to drop out,'" recalled Joe Shay, who did not come for the race.

Shay's physiotherapist in Flagstaff, Arizona—Phil Wharton—said that because Shay eventually responded to his regular massage therapy for fatigue and soreness after his tough workouts, they believed he was just exhausted from training.

"We'd have to work with him twice as long," Wharton said of the stretching and massage he did with Shay. "Maybe he wasn't getting the vascular flow."

"You could look at things that might have been red flags, but all of these things were normal to athletes training hard," said his wife, Alicia, a two-time 10,000 meter collegiate champion at Stanford. Together, the couple had been preparing for the trials at Northern Arizona University's Center for High Altitude Training.

His youngest brother, Stephan, had transferred to Brigham Young University on a track scholarship in September 2007, and he had visited Ryan and Alicia in Flagstaff prior to starting school. Stephan thought his brother seemed fatigued, but he understood why Shay would keep training hard.

"If you allow yourself to say that maybe you're working too hard, a lot of times you'll say that over and over again and then you're not going to work hard enough," Stephan said.

Days before the race in New York, however, Alicia said her husband was looking forward to the marathon, feeling prepared and calm. That was how he seemed the last time she saw him alive.

The Olympic trials course started at Rockefeller Center just past 7:35 a.m. on a damp, chilly Saturday. The runners made their way through Midtown Manhattan and into Central Park, where they would run four laps. Alicia had planned to dash between Central Park's east and west sides to catch a glimpse of Shay every three miles or so. Just past Mile Marker 5 at 8 a.m. on East Drive, she saw Ryan wearing bib No. 13. He was tucked in the back of the lead pack, which was running a somewhat slow 5-minute-per-mile pace.

"He was in a relaxed and rested state," Alicia said. "He was jogging almost. It looked like his body wasn't under any stress."

Shay passed the 15K mark (5.28 miles) at 8:02:54 a.m. By then, Alicia had left for her next planned viewing point, so she did not see Shay drift out of the pack about a minute later and crumple to the side of the road. According to the New York Road Runners' medical director, Dr. Lewis Maharam, Shay nearly fell onto two spectators. One was a former emergency medical technician and another was a rheumatology fellow who had just finished a residency in internal medicine. "At that point, he was breathing and had a pulse," Maharam said.

At 8:05:07 a.m., a New York police officer called in to the dispatch that a "sick runner" was down. It took nearly eight minutes for an ambulance to arrive after that initial call, at 8:12:57 a.m. By then, the two bystanders had already begun administering CPR.

When the paramedics from two ambulances arrived, they took over the CPR. Shay went into cardiac arrest at 8:15. On the way to Lenox Hill Hospital on 77th Street and Lexington Avenue, paramedics used defibrillators to shock him twice, but it was too late. The moment Alicia received a phone call from Wharton, Shay's physiotherapist, she sprinted out of the park to the hospital, four blocks away. She arrived at the emergency room as doctors were still working to revive Shay. He died at 8:45:59. Alicia, in utter shock, held her husband's still-warm body.

The athletes were out on the course at the time, about an hour away from finishing; they were unaware that something had gone dreadfully wrong. Ryan Hall, in front of the lead pack, never saw the ambulances behind him. At 25, running only his second marathon, Hall glided unchallenged over the final ten miles of Central Park's hills. With a broad smile, he high-fived fans as he approached the finish line and won in a trials record time of 2:09:02.

This was Hall's first exhilarating step in fulfilling an Olympic dream that had become an obsession for him since he was a teenager. Fifteen minutes after basking in his achievement, Hall was escorted to a room in Tavern on the Green with the other two Olympic qualifiers. There, Dathan Ritzenhein, the second-place finisher, turned to Hall and told him the terrible news.

At the same time, outside the room Ryan Hall's wife, Sara, also learned that Shay was dead. She had been a close friend of Alicia Shay's at Stanford, and was a bridesmaid at Alicia and Ryan's wedding only four months earlier. Ryan Hall had trained with Shay in Mammoth Lakes, California, and they had shared an easy friendship. The two young men were both coached by their fathers. They were guided by faith, and both had a penchant for running more than was asked of them. And of course, they shared a first name that would link them forever to this day. Hall would later say that friends and his family had called him, leaving urgent messages not of congratulations, but of concern. They feared he was the Ryan who had died.

Nobody would talk of much else but Ryan Shay that day. Ritzenhein was dazed and said that he could not possibly feel great about his own race. Brian Sell, the 29-year-old veteran who had his career breakthrough to finish third, dissolved in tears and held his head in his hands during the postrace press conference.

Meb Keflezighi, the silver medalist from the 2004 Athens Olympics and another former training partner of Shay's, finished eighth. He sobbed for fifteen minutes on the curb near the finish line when he was told the news. "The marathon is supposed to be about the disappointment of finishing fifth or sixth," Keflezighi said, his eyes bloodshot. He shook his head, adding: "It shouldn't be life or death."

Later that afternoon in a VIP room at Tavern on the Green, Joe Vigil, the U.S. marathon coach, sat stunned with 2004 Olympic bronze medalist, Deena Kastor, who had also trained with Shay. Dr. Dave Martin, the physiologist and historian, was in the room and would remember somebody mumbling the epitaph to the day.

"Quite a price to pick an Olympic team."

They all nodded in grief.

Martin added: "What price glory?"

Despite the somber mood, Martin said that no elite athlete came to him after Shay's death and wondered whether to stop running. "No one is afraid to toe the line and that's good. That would be overkill," said Martin, who works primarily with U.S. runners. "One thing elite athletes learn is to turn the page and move forward, be resilient. Things happen."

Paula Radcliffe would express her condolences in a press conference after the New York City Marathon the next day and say how his death put "everything into perspective a little bit." When asked a month later whether Shay's death would cause her to change her own workouts or if she thought vigorous training could be dangerous, even fatal, she would reply without hesitation.

"Honestly, no," Radcliffe would say. "The benefits of being fit and healthy are greater than the risks."

The race's medical director, Dr. Maharam, said his private practice was bombarded with about seventy-five calls from runners wondering if they could be susceptible to heart attacks. The following week Maharam would urge each of them to have a comprehensive physical, and if a heart murmur were found, he would refer them to a cardiologist.

Steve Gonzales, a first-time marathoner in town from Southern California to run the New York City Marathon, remembered laughing when his mother, Irene, told him before he left to be careful. He asked her what she meant and she responded: "Sometimes people's hearts don't take it that well."

He called her Saturday to acknowledge what happened to Shay and to reassure her that he would be fine. He would be.

But not everybody would be fine Sunday. Matthew P. Hardy, a 50-year-old research scientist in New York, would die at home three hours after finishing Sunday's Marathon. An autopsy would confirm a coronary artery blockage. He had just completed his twelfth New York City Marathon.

No participant has died in the New York City Marathon since 1994, when two runners, coincidentally both French-born, died of heart attacks after crossing the finish line. One man, who was living on Staten Island, was 27. The other man, who had traveled from France for the race, was 50.

The combined results of two recent studies of United States marathons show that approximately 1 in 100,000 runners died during marathons from 1976 to 2004. "Anybody who thinks there is zero risk to anything is wrong," said cardiologist Paul Thompson, Director of Preventive Cardiology at Hartford Hospital. "People have to realize there are risks doing competitive sports. But if you live a life of no chances, you've not lived."

Shay's unrelenting work ethic would endure as his public legacy, even as his family and friends found their own way to come to terms with his death. Hall would cut out the picture from the

Sunday *New York Times* that showed him standing next to Shay on the starting line. That morning Hall had been caught up in his stretching and rushed late to the start, asking Shay if he could squeeze in next to him. Hall would carry that picture in his bible as a bookmarker and a powerful reminder: "Life is precious," Hall would say at the London Marathon in April 2008, where he turned in an astounding 2:06:17 performance for fifth place to prepare him for the Beijing Olympics.

Stephan would memorialize his older brother by getting a tattoo on his left thigh that was identical to Ryan's—the family Irish crest, in blue and yellow. But he would not undergo any heart tests before his indoor track season.

"I know it's something I need to do," Stephan will say in February 2008 when he runs in New York at an indoor collegiate meet. "I don't know if it would make a difference. If they told me I had an enlarged heart and something could happen, I don't know that I'd stop running. Running's not my life, but I put a lot of time and effort into it."

That weekend, Stephan would make a point of visiting the spot in Central Park where his brother collapsed. On a flat stone, someone had scratched SHAY in white block letters, along with Ryan's life dates: 79–07. The stone is all that remains of a makeshift memorial that appeared in the days after his death.

That February day, Stephan would see a group of cyclists going up the hill and could hear their conversation. "That's where Ryan passed away," he would hear one cyclist say to his friends. Stephan would feel gratified they remembered his brother and would be comforted by the park's setting.

"I imagined him running down the hill and seeing the city in the background," Stephan will say. "It's a beautiful spot."

Alicia might visit the spot someday, if she can muster the

strength. New York was where she and Ryan met. The Road Runners' chief executive, Mary Wittenberg, had brought Alicia in for the 2005 Marathon on a recruiting mission. The night after the race, Alicia met Shay at Rosie O'Grady's bar in Manhattan. Shay had finished in eighteenth place that day, suffering through a foot injury, but the pain and disappointment dissolved as soon as he started talking to Alicia. They were married less than two years later.

Alicia would continue training, knowing where one day she might best honor her husband's memory. "I always wanted to run the New York City Marathon," Alicia will say in February 2008. "No—I want to win the New York City Marathon one day. To me, it's like the ultimate marathon."

25

THE RACE MUST GO ON

Mile 25, East Drive to Central Park South

Jennifer Malone can hear the cheers drifting from the finish line over on the west side of the Park as the course turns uphill again past the boathouse and Mile Marker 25. As much as her legs are aching to stop, her heart wants to stay suspended in the reverie. Malone can feel her husband, Clint, as if he were still next to her, just like he was until the moment he died.

Perhaps more than anyone else today, Jennifer Malone can understand Alicia Shay's anguish, her disbelief and her sudden emptiness.

Clint Malone had always been the cautious one. "Mr. Safety," Malone called her husband. He was not a runner, but he would often help Malone train for a marathon by riding his bicycle alongside her when she ran. When Malone had told him how New York would be the ultimate marathon experience, Clint enlisted a friend who worked for ING, the Marathon's title sponsor, to secure an entry.

The race was just three weeks away when the couple, who resided in Vero Beach, Florida, visited Clint's parents in Panama City Beach over the Columbus Day weekend. Jennifer and Clint Malone left the house at 4:45 a.m. on that Saturday, October 13, Clint riding his father's beach cruiser beside or right behind his running wife, depending on traffic. He had mapped out a safe route the night before, but at the last minute he changed his mind, thinking the new route would have more sidewalks. "He would always say, 'It's not that I don't trust you; I just don't trust the people in that car,'" Malone recalled.

The morning was cool—57 degrees—and perfect for a 23-mile training run. "I just know you're going to have race weather like this for New York," Clint told his wife that morning, and he would be correct again.

For the first hour, the couple talked and laughed and made future plans. Clint reminisced about his high school years in Panama City Beach. They both expressed how grateful they were to have found each other at the University of Florida, how thankful they were to have two healthy children, Jackson, nearly three, and Mary Kathryn, seventeen months. They were fully in love, appreciating this time together. As Malone would say later, "Thank God for that hour. It was one of the best hours in our life."

The couple stopped to use the bathroom at a convenience store and then got back on the road, following a stretch where the sidewalk ended. As they made a turn, Clint saw Pineapple Willy's, a restaurant he used to love, and he promised to take his wife there if his parents would babysit that night.

"Traffic's picking up, honey," Clint warned Malone from a few feet back, "make sure . . ."

Malone thinks those were his last words. She cannot quite remember, considering what followed. "Seconds later, my husband and the bike were flying past me," she said.

Malone took off on a frantic sprint, screaming, waving her hands, trying to catch the sports utility vehicle—was it maroon or white?—speeding away. When she finally found her husband, 300 yards away, he was not breathing and his head was gushing blood. His shoes were strewn on the lawn. So was one of his bicycle tires. The family in the house near where he landed heard Malone's shrill screams and rushed to call for help. But Malone knew instantly that it was bad. She put her hand on Clint's stomach and felt that he was not breathing.

Later, when the paramedics motioned her to the front of the ambulance after five minutes of working on him, she saw the white sheet covering Clint. Her hysterics turned to shock and back to hysterics again.

Three days after Clint died, the driver of that maroon Ford Bronco turned himself in. Jeremy Matthew Hunt, 20, worked at a bar down the street; Panama City Beach police believed that alcohol could have been a factor in the hit-and-run. He was immediately charged with leaving the scene of an accident involving death. By the end of January, Hunt would also be charged with vehicular homicide and tampering with evidence. By May, the charge would be adjusted to DUI manslaughter, since, according to Jennifer Malone, there was video footage of Hunt's drinking that evening in the bar where he had worked.

Hunt had struck Clint Malone, going what police would record as between 38 and 47 miles an hour in a 30-mile-per-hour zone. Hunt had removed the front grille of his vehicle, which showed the damage from the collision. Malone dreaded going through a criminal trial. She wanted retribution, but she desperately wanted to be able to move on.

For days after the funeral, she could not eat or get out of bed. She did not know if she could move her feet. She never wanted to run again.

One morning in the week after Clint's death, her son, Jackson, walked into her bedroom. "Mommy," he said. "Do you think you could get up today?"

She smiled at him. "You got it, buddy."

Malone forced herself to walk out of the bedroom and then run again, realizing she had to eat properly if she wanted to fuel her body in order to complete the New York City Marathon. She continued training with two friends, Janae Collins and Jeri Lynn Kranze, because she was determined to honor her husband's memory. "Clint was so supportive. He did everything he could to get me into it," she said. "I had to do it."

Today, the three women are dressed in identical green tank tops, with a picture of Clint Malone on the back, his arms in the shape of a V for victory, and the words, In Loving Memory. On the front of her shirt, Malone puts her name and the numeral 3, Clint's special code number for her.

Until Mile 25, she can barely wipe the smile off her face. She is buoyed by the memory of her father, who had died two years ago and loved New York. But ultimately, she makes this Marathon a celebration of Clint's life: "He worked hard, played hard, lived hard and loved hard."

So she runs hard.

Malone basks in the comfort of 39,000 runners on the Verrazano-Narrows Bridge, awestruck by the fireboats spewing red, white and blue in the harbor. The fans lining the course amaze and uplift her, and the sight of Manhattan skyscrapers from the Queensboro Bridge makes her giddy. She had never run in Central Park before, and when she gets there, the hills are a surprise. The smile fades.

Her brother, sisters and friends are all waiting at the finish line. The day before, a friend came to the city from Connecticut and told Malone how her sister had known Ryan Shay at Notre Dame.

"I thought, Here's this guy in incredible shape," Malone said. "He's just starting his life with his wife. I was so sad for his family."

In less than two miles, Malone will feel elated when volunteers lay the medal over her neck, with ING's orange, blue and white colors on its lanyard.

"Gator colors—Clint would have loved it," she will think, recalling their University of Florida days.

Seconds later, though, the exhilaration will drain and the one person she wants to hug most will not be there.

That night, her family will take her out to dinner and uplift her again. It is an ongoing process of recovery. Her brother will give her an official Marathon T-shirt with the words: "I finished what I started."

Malone will be comforted, at least temporarily. "That's the theme of my life," she will say. "I felt like I had him with me."

The race must go on. And here in the rolling downhill stretches of Central Park, the women's professional race turns into a game of cat and mouse—while another cat watches.

Radcliffe and Wami speed down the hill known among runners and cyclists as Cat Hill, named after the life-size bronze statue of a panther perched on a rock that juts out over East Park Drive, at about 78th Street. The sculpture, titled "Still Hunt," was created in 1883 by Edward Kemeys, who became the country's foremost bronze sculptor of animals.

The menacing cat has been known to startle runners, but nothing seems to get to Radcliffe today. She takes advantage of the downhill to break from Wami again after passing a large Union Jack flag held by two fans. She has a good seven-foot lead over Wami just past Mile Marker 25 when they reach the bottom of the hill.

Wami still has a blank look on her face. A war rages in her stomach, upset from the small amount of pasta she ate in the morning and the energy drinks she ingested. Still, she looks like she is cruising along on a Sunday run in the mountains above Addis Ababa.

Wami may have shown her vulnerability, but Radcliffe has not seen it. Wami again pulls within footsteps of Paula as the pair makes a sharp right turn out of the park and onto the straightaway of Central Park South.

A little less than one mile remains.

By the time Martin Lel and Abderrahim Goumri turn on to Central Park South, nothing has changed. They are still locked, stride for elongated stride—Lel on the left, Goumri on the right.

Goumri, however, almost did not make it to this point, let alone arrive in New York. His story is one that is becoming increasingly familiar for foreign athletes: visa problems.

By late July, he and his Pittsburgh-based agent, John Nubani, had already started the process to obtain a visa for Goumri to travel from Morocco to New York in November. They enlisted the help of his shoe sponsor, Nike, to expedite a P–1 visa, the type issued for professional athletes and entertainers. United States immigration procedures have become more stringent, expensive and cumbersome with background checks since the terrorist attacks of September 11, 2001, and some foreign athletes have had difficulty obtaining visas to compete in the United States. (Salina Kosgei, of Kenya, was not able to secure her visa in time and withdrew from this year's race.)

A process that might have taken only thirty days under the old, expedited system dragged out for Goumri. Nubani had to file extensive documentation about Goumri's athletic achievements and solicit a signature from an official with USA Track & Field, in addition to having Nike sponsor the visa petition. An extra $1,000 was required for the expedition process.

But one week before the New York City Marathon, Goumri still did not have his visa. He spent an anxious five days traveling from the high-altitude training center in Ifrane to the Moroccan capital of Rabat and then to the U.S. Consulate in Casablanca. Officials with the Consulate told him he needed a formal interview. But according to Nubani, once the U.S. Bureau of Citizenship and Immigration Services (a division of the Department of Homeland Security) sent Goumri's approval notice on letterhead via e-mail, the U.S. Consulate in Casablanca then required the original letter.

By the time Goumri got the letter—express global mail took four days—and delivered it to the consulate, it was Wednesday before the Marathon. He was told to return the next morning in Casablanca for official documentation. Goumri finally received his visa at 10 a.m. Thursday, Moroccan time. His flight was at noon out of Casablanca Mohammed V Airport. He told the taxi driver to step on it.

Goumri arrived in New York, grateful, at 6 p.m. Thursday.

"I think if you have problems before the race that can be good, because then you are not thinking too much about the race," Goumri said, laughing in the comfort of hindsight.

Since athletes taper usually two weeks before a marathon, the traveling and uncertainty that week were nerve-racking but manageable for Goumri. He had already dealt with another more intense disruption in his training. From September 13 to October 12, the prime preparation period for marathoners, Goumri fasted with his fellow Muslim runners during the day in observance of Ramadan. They would train early in the morning after a meal and then again in the evening after breaking the fast. Although Goumri has fasted during Ramadan throughout his career, this was the first time he did so while training for a marathon.

"I am Muslim and I believe this is important," he said. "This is my life."

Goumri and Lel are feeling each other out for the right moment to break, running just under a 5-minute-per-mile pace in the shadow of towering prewar apartments, the famous Plaza Hotel (now approximately half hotel rooms and half condominiums), and tourist attractions like Mickey Mantle's restaurant on Central Park South. This has been the corridor for so many of the Marathon's defining duels and dramas. But at Seventh Avenue, two blocks from where the runners turn back into the park, one solo sideline act steals the show.

Sensing the pain the runners feel in the last half-mile of the race, NYPD officer John Codiglia makes it his job to lighten the mood. Standing on the far corner of Seventh Avenue and Central Park South, outside the New York Athletic Club, Codiglia brandishes a bullhorn below his thick mustache. A burly operations commander of Patrol Borough Manhattan South—from 59th Street down to Battery Park City—Codiglia cheers the runners and marshals them back into the park and toward the finish line.

He shouts jokes and encouragement on his bullhorn:

"What took you so long? I've been waiting for you all day!"

"You didn't come to this event to start the race; you come to finish!"

And, for the Italian runners he spots: *"Forzo ragazzo! Molto lontano a Roma!"* (Rough translation: "You go, boy! It sure is a long way to Rome!")

Over the course of six hours, he stands with his bullhorn on the corner. He likes to vary his routine for the runners. "Anything," he said, "to take their minds off running."

Codiglia wants to be a part of their journey, even if they are so dazed by then they may not remember it.

Codiglia remembers his own journey, even though it was a half century ago. It began in Trieste, Italy, in 1956. He was 10 years old. His father had died, and his mother, Ermenia, decided to bring him and his older sister, Adriana, to New York. They arrived safely, but as he likes to recount, their belongings did not. They were on the SS *Andrea Doria*, the ocean liner that sank off Nantucket following a collision with the eastbound MS *Stockholm*, another ocean liner.

"My most favorite red sweater, the one with the reindeer, lies some 245 feet off the coast of Massachusetts," Codiglia said.

He joined the police department in 1969. Now 61, he puts a little extra oomph into his calls this year since it could likely be his last Marathon; rules state he must retire from the police department in his sixty-third year, which officially begins when he turns 62. Codiglia says he is hoping to come back to work the Marathon as a volunteer since he has worked it for twenty-eight years, thirteen on this, his favorite corner.

At 8 a.m., he gathers the troops from his section, some 115 strong, and gives them a short lecture on the history of the Marathon and on how the police force can enhance the runners' experience.

"This is an opportunity for New York City and its residents to showcase New York City hospitality and the diversity represented," he says. "Hopefully they'll have an impression of a city that might have its problems, but overall it's working."

One Marathon Sunday stands out to him as an example of how a police officer helped rescue the race. Runners, he explains, are in a trancelike state, just trying to find ways to overcome the pain when they reach the final half-mile of the course.

In 1994, German Silva and Benjamin Paredes, both from Mexico, were racing neck and neck for first place as they stormed onto Central Park South flanked by a motorcycle escort and a camera truck. They had a half mile to go in the race when Silva strangely turned right, one block earlier than he was supposed to—away from a shocked Paredes. Silva had mistakenly followed the press vehicle, which was taking a shortcut to the finish line.

Silva took twelve steps into the park and, with a policeman trying to wave him back, he suddenly realized there were no more fans lining the course. As Silva retraced his steps, his horror fueled his adrenaline, and he ultimately passed Paredes for the victory.

Codiglia was in charge of the officer who waved Silva back on course. "I remember talking to the officer, telling him, 'You helped this man win the race by redirecting him,'" Codiglia recalled.

Silva returned to win the Marathon again in 1995, this time without the unscheduled detour. But to this day, Silva cannot live down his mistake. He still laughs about it when the runners he now coaches in Mexico mention it.

"Many people remember the wrong-way winner," he said.

This year, he helped prepare thirty runners at his training facility in San Luis Potosi, in the north of Mexico, to run the New York City Marathon. He also did some "guest coaching" in New York for a promising runner from Fred's Team, Matthew Farver. A dancer in the musical *Mamma Mia!*, Farver, 31, today will finish in a remarkable 2:52:32 in only his second attempt, two years removed from overcoming testicular cancer.

Silva's dramatic victories in New York were the last from a Mexican runner before the Kenyans began dominating; even now, he sees how his success helped popularize the marathon in Mexico.

"It has become so much a part of their lifestyle," he said. "These are people who are looking for something to make sense for their lives."

As much as Silva has become a folk hero in New York City Marathon lore for his literal comeback victory in 1994, that one race held a more personal significance for him. Silva was able to take his winnings and install electricity in his father's remote village of El Tecomate, in Mexico. Silva made appearances throughout Mexico in the months after the Marathon, not realizing how sick his father, Agapito, had become. Silva decided to live and train in El Tecomate as soon as a relative told him, and he spent an emotional last few months of his father's life with him. "He became my biggest fan," Silva said.

Agapito died from cancer in June 1995, inspiring Silva to his second victory that November. In this race, today and every year, it seems, life and death work together as training partners.

26

MAKING THE MOVE

Mile 26, Central Park South to West Drive

Gete Wami has been staring at Paula Radcliffe's back for 26 miles. Wami has not come to New York to sightsee. And she has not run the better part of five boroughs only to be content with a consolation prize. Although—it is one heck of a bonanza. No, she will not think about the $500,000 that waits for her as long as she finishes ahead of Jelena Prokopcuka, who is a good three minutes behind her. Wami is a competitor, still, and in her thirty-third career showdown with Radcliffe, she has one move left.

If these two were running this final stretch—a little less than a half mile—on the flat track, Wami would likely have the advantage. She has surged past Radcliffe in two notable 10,000 meter races, and in virtually every cross-country race of their careers.

But here on the road, where the final 400 yards in Central Park are uphill on asphalt, this is decidedly Radcliffe's domain. And both women know it.

Radcliffe's stranglehold on her road competitors is perhaps more psychological than physical. Her success begets confidence and vice versa. Three days before the race, Radcliffe came to the Columbus

Circle entrance to the park and fiercely practiced her strides to the finish line for muscle memory.

Wami went for her own preparatory runs in the park. But the night before the race, she and her husband, Getaneh Tessema, went for an evening stroll along Sixth Avenue; she was that relaxed.

Radcliffe has not looked back once at Wami all day today. Until now. For the first time, on Central Park South, Radcliffe quickly jerks her head over her left shoulder. Wami is five feet behind her. And gaining.

Just past Seventh Avenue, Wami pulls even to Radcliffe's left shoulder and, for the first time all race, is three feet astride of her. Then, suddenly, Wami surges ahead—one yard and then another. Wami should be feeling free, should be getting that rush of adrenaline to carry her into the straightaway. But where is it?

She searches and finds nothing in the tank. Nothing but bile.

Wami is trying to squeeze one last anguished drop of energy from her souring stomach and her leaden muscles. Her legs have checked out, returning to the Brandenburg Gate, the scene of her Berlin victory 35 days ago.

Even she cannot sell this surge.

Wami's one and only challenge of the day is significant enough to ignite Radcliffe's competitive flame, which has been lying dormant for two marathon-less years.

I'm not giving up now, Radcliffe thinks.

She came into the day believing that if all went well, she would likely make her decisive move around the final 500 meters. She also promised herself that she would cover any surge a rival made during the race. There are 869 meters left in this race, a little over a half mile.

OK, Radcliffe thinks, *I will just make my move a little earlier.*

With ferocious efficiency, Radcliffe eradicates an eight-second blip of doubt and rockets past Wami. Wami immediately decelerates to a resigned jog, to the point where she appears to be running in reverse.

Race over.

Wami watches as Radcliffe storms toward her second New York City Marathon title. The consolation prize awaits.

For the second time in a major city marathon this year, the men's race has come down to Martin Lel and Abderrahim Goumri. This is the first New York City Marathon Lel has been healthy enough to participate since he won in 2003. He has had few problems since winning the 2007 London Marathon in April.

Today, he has but one hill left in the race—the slight climb to the finish line that looms only a right turn away. Goumri has run a smart race until this point. He was careful to stay behind Hendrick Ramaala and Lel when they surged in Brooklyn and then again on First Avenue. On Fifth Avenue, perhaps Goumri was too careful by staying with Lel, rather than taking the lead himself.

Now the Kenyan has the Moroccan upstart just where he wants him. Lel has the benefit of experience, just as he did in London where he knew the course. No matter how much Goumri discussed the hills on the course with his coach, the 2000 New York winner, Abdelkhader el-Mouaziz, he had memorized neither the tangents nor the other nuances of the final stretch.

Lel can think back to 2003 when he was running with his countryman, Rodgers Rop, in this same stretch on Central Park South. That year, after they reentered the park, Lel sprinted past Rop in the final 200 yards to claim his first Marathon title.

When Lel returned home victorious from that race, however, his neighbors kept calling him for assistance. He felt he could not refuse. The constant supplication was, at times, a distraction for a generous man who prefers to keep a low profile.

Lel was grateful to escape before this year's marathon to the western mountains of Italy so that he could train in seclusion with his coaches, Dr. Gabriela Rosa and Claudio Berardelli. In the thin air, Lel felt as if he could finally exhale.

"There was no pressure," he said. "Your mind is only on training."

To strengthen his legs for New York, Berardelli had Lel run a series of uphill sprints that also alleviated the pressure on his feet. "That running helps the legs be elastic so they can accept any kind of training," Berardelli said.

But he found Lel's mind to be even more resilient. "I am dealing with one of the strongest athletes mentally, ever," Berardelli added.

Today in the final straightaway of Central Park South, Lel gains momentum, already plotting how to take out his rival. He turns right around Columbus Circle and heads back into the park. Instead of going the way of inertia, however, and floating to the right with the road's curve, Lel dips his shoulder and veers left toward the opposite curb, completely blocking Goumri from passing him.

Goumri is directly behind Lel and to his right. By the time Goumri figures out how to counter this move and tries to go the other way around his rival, Lel takes off.

Twenty yards into Central Park, Lel separates himself from his upstart competitor for the second consecutive marathon.

Lel passes another Kenyan to his left. It is the tiny Tegla Loroupe, who returned to her country after winning in 1994 and 1995 to fund running programs for girls in Kenya. Now she runs marathons for fun and today will finish in eighth place, just about 20 minutes behind the leaders. Lel is carrying on her philanthropic legacy in a more subtle way.

He turns his head back to spot Goumri. Thirty yards or so

remain. Lel is not taking any chances. The man with the best kick in the sport prepares to finish with a flourish.

The 26.2 mile marathon distance—the point two equaling 385 yards—came to be because of the British royal family and their tinkering at the 1908 London Olympics. The first three Olympic marathons were about 25 miles—the approximate distance Pheidippides ran from the town of Marathon to Athens. But Great Britain's Princess of Wales and her mother-in-law, Queen Alexandra, had other ideas. In 1908, the princess requested that the start be moved to Windsor Castle so that she and her children might be able to see the runners start, thus stretching the course to 26 miles. But Queen Alexandra, who was to be in the Olympic Stadium, had one more idea. She requested that once the runners enter the stadium, they complete nearly one full lap before finishing the race in front of the royal box. Hence—the extra 385 yards.

Mile marker 26—displayed in a large overhead banner as the runners reenter Central Park—advertises that the end is near. At this point, however, there are some who might be feeling suspiciously better than they should. Bandits. The newest incarnations of Rosie Ruiz.

Before Ruiz infamously scandalized the running community by jumping into the 1980 Boston Marathon at the end of the race and crossing the finish line first among 448 women, she did her test run (and ride) in the October 1979 New York City Marathon. Her time of 2:56:29 there had qualified her to run the Boston Marathon.

But a day after her "victory," in Boston, Susan Morrow, a New York freelance photographer, was moved to tell her story about Ruiz's participation in the New York Marathon to the *New York Times*'s Neil Amdur. Amdur, in Boston to cover the marathon, had reported the inconsistencies and skepticism surrounding Ruiz's run there.

Morrow said that in New York she had ridden the subway with Ruiz from West Fourth Street in Greenwich Village to Columbus Circle. Ruiz told her she had dropped out due to a sprained ankle after 10 miles. Morrow and Ruiz walked to the finish line. But because Ruiz was still wearing her number, she was able to walk inside the course barricades. She claimed she had been injured, and New York officials recorded her time. Suddenly, Ruiz had finished the 1979 New York City Marathon as the twenty-fourth fastest woman.

After Ruiz's race in Boston, Fred Lebow immediately checked the video tape and race-sponsored photography from the previous October. He then used Morrow's account to supplement that information, determining that Ruiz had not crossed the finish line in New York. He disqualified her from the New York race. Boston soon invalidated her victory there. More ignominy followed.

In 1982, Ruiz was arrested in New York on charges of forgery and grand larceny; she spent one week in jail and was sentenced to five years' probation. Eighteen months later she was arrested in Miami on charges of selling cocaine, as part of an all-woman cocaine ring. She was sentenced to three years' probation in Florida.

As records would show, Ruiz had gained entry to New York through a special exemption from the Achilles Track Club because she supposedly had terminal brain cancer. It was a sad footnote considering her cheating—and that she continued to deny it—devastated Fred Lebow, who would die of that particular cancer.

"It was in his soul," Amdur said. "I don't think Fred ever recovered from it."

But Lebow made sure his race recovered as the New York Road Runners tightened the monitoring system in order to maintain the

Marathon's integrity. Since 1997, runners have worn electronic-chip timers on their shoes, making the bandit-chasing business significantly easier. Later, timing pads were placed at 5 kilometer intervals to make the monitoring more sophisticated.

Tom Kelley, the Road Runners' director of race-scoring operations, searches the data for anomalies after the race. If runners miss a pad or multiple pads or have an unusual surge in pace between markers, Road Runners sends them a letter allowing them to come clean. Kelley also uses the event-photography company, brightroom, which captures everybody on course wearing a number, to cross-reference the suspicious runners.

In 2007, Road Runners will disqualify twenty-three runners for cheating. Only three are women. None is the actor Katie Holmes.

Despite furious Internet discussion that questioned the authenticity of her race, Holmes, the wife of Tom Cruise, did finish, according to Kelley and his assistant, Jud Santos. They carefully analyzed each of her split times. She hit every 5K timing pad. Kelley acknowledged, however, that the Road Runners' bandit chasers— volunteers out on the course to catch the garden variety bandit, such as people who run without proper bib numbers or chips—did miss one of Holmes's running partners, who wore a bib from 2003. Kelley found that strange since the Road Runners had granted four official bibs to her team before the race.

Jodi Richard, chief of the volunteer "bandit catchers" for the last twelve years, finds herself distracted during the time Holmes and her crew come running by Columbus Circle on the way to the finish line. She is dumbstruck by a man who somehow gained access to the course dressed as a gypsy and pushing a baby carriage. He angrily tries to convince Richard on Central Park South that he has been in the race from the start. Runners pushing baby joggers are not even allowed in this race. On the top of this man's baby carriage sit a parrot and a toy poodle. She tells him to get lost—and off the course.

Richard's group will catch approximately fifty people trying to sneak to the finish line today without a bib or a chip. And they will stop hundreds more as a precaution.

When he reenters the park, Harrie Bakst has no idea why someone is running after him and shouting. It is about 4:30 p.m., and the temperature has dropped to the low 50s. Harrie has put back on the olive green long-sleeved wicking shirt he had taken on and off throughout the course. And now it is covering his bib number.

A bandit chaser hunts him down from behind and shouts to him to flash his number. Harrie has to stop, turn around and lift up his outer shirt, which causes him to lose his momentum completely, just as the course turns uphill again.

With but 500 meters to go, Harrie must prove once again that he belongs.

26.2

REASONS AND REVELATIONS

The Finish Line

If the starting village in Staten Island resembles an eclectic carnival and the entire New York City Marathon a five-borough parade, then Central Park's finish line is like Mardi Gras—unwinding in its final, bedraggled hour. By the time the runners reenter the park, they are more than ready for the Marathon to end.

Only two women and two men actually break the tape—in the elite wheelchair and running divisions. For the rest of the field, the real celebration has already occurred, step by step, with surprises unfolding on every block.

Today they spill across the finish line alone or they hold the hands of old and new friends. Their colorful costumes and personalized outfits from the morning are faded, their lips caked in salt, their tops clinging to dried sweat—a grime scene of exhausted elation.

A pair of platinum-haired women holding Canadian flags cross the line, followed by a crying one-armed woman wearing a Superman costume, complete with red cape. A 7-foot runner from Holland wears an orange wig and a T-shirt that promotes the obvious: Tall Man.

Finishers stagger toward volunteers waiting to hang a medal on their necks. On the front of the people's bronze medal, two runners in Central Park raise their arms at the finish line, in relief. On the back of the medal, Alberto Salazar has provided the inscription this year: A Triumph of the Will over All Limits.

They are appropriate words for the 2007 New York City Marathon, especially coming from a man who dodged death only months earlier. The will to live and the will to win carry 38,676 today to the limit and beyond. But for the 1,129 who drop out along the way, even will is not enough.

"If you can make it here, you can make it anywhere. New York, New York," sing-songs the back of the elite medals in gold, silver and bronze. On the front, the Verrazano-Narrows Bridge rises majestically. The day has come full circle.

People start for a reason; they finish with a revelation.

It might be an affirmation: *I can do this.*

It might be a proclamation: *I'll never do this again!* (Grete Waitz and Lance Armstrong both said this after their first marathons in New York. Never trust a postrace proclamation.)

The revelation might be a declaration: *I survived.*

Or it might come in the form of a promise: *Same time, next year: the first Sunday in November.*

For everyone from the professional to the recreational runner, the finish line clock marks a day's work and validates the journey.

1:52:38—

When Edith Hunkeler climbs toward the finish line, she is all alone, as she has been in the final three miles. Hunkeler wins her race when she first turns into Central Park at 90th Street. After a quick look behind her shoulder, she sees Great Britain's Shelly Woods in her draft as well as the defending champion and Illinois University student, Amanda McGrory, a bit farther behind.

"Let's go now," Hunkeler says to herself. She pumps her arms and spins her wheels into overdrive, never looking back again.

This is why she rehabilitated after the second accident in her life—a gruesome crash while competing at the 2006 World Championships—and would not accept the answer the doctor gave her. Her career is not over, as he said; rather it is just beginning again. Hunkeler breaks her own course record, which she set in 2005, by 51 seconds.

Wheeling across the finish line, she pumps her arms, and buries her head into her knees. She does not know whether to scream for joy or cry. She does both.

Her coach, André Fries, runs out to the road beyond the finish line and hugs her while she is still sitting in her chair.

Hunkeler finishes about twenty minutes after Kurt Fearnley of Australia, who has repeated his victory as the men's wheelchair champion, with a time of 1:33:58. Fearnley finishes 1 minute and 10 seconds ahead of Krige Schabort and more than four minutes slower than his own course record.

Hunkeler's margin of victory over Shelly Woods is 1 minute, 41 seconds. For breaking the women's course record, she wins a $5,000 bonus to go with her first-place check of $12,500.

"This year was so special—the first after the accident," she says.

How special?

"I can't explain it," Hunkeler will say later. "I couldn't sleep for three days."

2:23:09—

Paula Radcliffe does not dare look back, fearing that Gete Wami will run past her to the tape. She has sunk completely into a trance, not even hearing British race announcer Ian Brooks shout, "Here she comes! Paula Radcliffe!" with a familiar accent.

Usually, Radcliffe helps overcome the pain of a marathon's final miles by counting her steps or repeating a mantra. And in her first marathon in more than two years, she does have pain; the unfamiliar pounding causes her legs to feel as though they are dragging 20-pound weights.

When Wami was right behind her as motivation, Radcliffe did not need a mantra. Until the end. Once she passes Wami and makes her charge up the final hill of Central Park, only then does she start the incantation.

"Isla, Isla, Isla," Radcliffe chants, as her lips form the words and her head bobs frantically back and forth.

"Isla, Isla, Isla," she repeats, as she draws closer to the reunion with her infant daughter.

A few feet away from the finish, Radcliffe can finally sense she is alone. She throws her arms out to her sides—there is not a superfluous fold of skin on her body—and breaks the tape. A split second later, Radcliffe stops her watch on instinct: 2:23:09, beating her 2004 victory here by one second.

She takes the Union Jack from Mary Wittenberg, drapes it around her bony shoulders and asks the race director in wide-eyed concern what happened to Wami. Radcliffe thinks Wami was right behind her, as she was throughout the race. She worries. Perhaps Wami was accosted? Maybe something happened to her like what happened in the men's marathon at the Athens Olympics when a defrocked priest entered the course and tackled the Brazilian runner, Lima de Vanderlei.

It is a strange, albeit caring thought from Radcliffe. It is the kind of thought so disconnected from reality, that it shows just how little blood is circulating to Radcliffe's brain. She could not yet process the magnitude of her throwdown move.

Wittenberg laughs and reassures Radcliffe that Wami is on her way.

Twenty-three seconds later, when Wami crosses the line, Radcliffe bends her body in half to hug the woman who clipped her heels at least twice and who drafted off of her for all but six seconds of this 26.2-mile race.

They kiss each other on both cheeks and walk, each dazed, around the finish area.

Wami wobbles to the side of the road and dry heaves for a minute. Her stomach is rebelling, but it has no ammunition.

Radcliffe's husband, Gary Lough, is all charged up behind the barricades, bouncing on his heels just after Radcliffe crosses the finish line.

"She wasn't going to lose to Gete," Lough says, shaking his head. "She remembers Belgium."

Before Radcliffe moved to the marathon distance, she had been plagued by her failures to close out her opponents—especially Wami. At the 2001 IAAF World Cross-Country Championships in Belgium, she beat Wami one day and lost to her the next. But since 2002, when Radcliffe started running marathons, she has locked into a 26.2-mile comfort zone. Today marks the seventh victory in the eight marathons she has started, the one exception being when she dropped out of the 2004 Olympics.

"This is very much my event," Radcliffe will say matter-of-factly. "This is where I hold the most cards, technically. I think that gives me more confidence."

Radcliffe picks up a $170,000 winner's check, including the $40,000 time bonus for going faster than 2:23:30. She has already earned more than twice that in appearance fees and negotiated bonuses for this race.

Immediately after the race, reporters already start asking her about the Olympics in Beijing, nine months away. The climate there promises to be insufferable, they say—hotter, more humid and with worse pollution than in Athens—all conditions that would not seem to favor Radcliffe. No matter how obvious it seems, she denies that she feels pressure for Olympic redemption.

"It's totally different this time," Radcliffe says. "I feel like I'm starting with a clean slate. You don't carry any baggage from one to the next."

Except that she will, indeed, carry familiar baggage—of the heaviest kind.

Weeks after New York, Radcliffe will discover that the pain she felt in her feet in the final miles—the third toe in her right foot, especially—will turn into a full-fledged injury. She has run today's Marathon with the joint in her third toe locked up, only she did not realize it at the time. During the final miles of the race Radcliffe could not distinguish one pain from another; her legs and back and virtually everything else hurt.

It is only when she and Lough look at the video that they discern a slight limp; they notice she is not able to push off the right foot and is not using it properly. No wonder she had no power to pass Wami early in the park today. Radcliffe would rest, be refitted for orthotics and start training again in Albuquerque in February, but the injury would flare again and damage tendons in the second and third toes. Radcliffe would withdraw from the April 2008 London Marathon, only to resume training a few weeks later, despite a different pain. In May 2008, she would learn that she suffered a stress fracture in her left femur that would put her Beijing Olympics hopes in serious jeopardy.

Through the emotional, vicious cycle of training, victory and injury, it is her daughter who keeps her grounded. This is the kind of baggage that Radcliffe enjoys carrying: baby bottles, diapers, Dora the Explorer bags, DVDs, jumpers, strollers and tiny sneakers.

Now in the finish line area, Radcliffe takes Isla from her husband and bounces her in the pink dress that Wittenberg bought for her. The cameras are clicking.

The picture of Radcliffe holding Isla will be broadcast around the world, on front pages back in Great Britain, in magazines, on souvenir photos. She will be hailed as a medical marvel, returning nine months after childbirth. Not only did she win the New York City Marathon, she led for all but 10 seconds, obliterating the field.

Radcliffe does not see that she accomplished anything extraordinary. Rather, she finds fault in her return to racing.

"I thought it took me a long time to get back," Radcliffe will say two months after the race. "It should have taken me less time than it did. It took me too long."

Radcliffe admits that her life is much richer and more satisfying now that she has Isla to delight her. But that should not mean that she changed as an athlete.

"It took me by surprise a little, the impact it had back home," she will say. "It never crossed my mind that I couldn't do it."

2:23:32—

Gete Wami, as if out for a noontime playdate with other mothers in Central Park, asks Radcliffe if she can hold Isla at the finish line. Radcliffe hands her daughter to her rival, completing the symmetry. Six hours earlier, Wami's husband Getaneh Tessema had held Isla after the women boarded the bus for Staten Island.

In retrospect, Wami and Tessema will agree that perhaps she should have saved her one passing move until a little bit later, until there were maybe only 400 meters to go. But at the time, Wami rationalized that she was testing Radcliffe, hoping Radcliffe would not have the stamina to stay with her. Wami did not anticipate that she, herself, would run out of energy so soon.

If Wami does not look like a woman defeated that is because she is actually the day's biggest money winner. Her gamble on Central Park South cost her nothing at all. Because she won the Berlin Marathon twice in two years and finished second in London and now second in New York in 2007, Gete will collect $500,000 from the World Marathon Majors series. It is a winner-take-all prize.

For finishing second in the New York City Marathon, she will collect $65,000 plus a time bonus of $35,000. She misses an additional $5,000 time bonus by just two seconds—not too costly, considering her windfall.

Monday afternoon at the World Marathon Majors awards luncheon, in a well-intentioned speech of painfully halting English, Wami will thank all the people who have supported her—her agents, her husband and "my daughter, Eva, who has been an inspiration for me."

She says she plans to give money to orphanages in her home city of Addis Ababa. In the ensuing months after the Marathon, Wami and her husband will look into buying a plot of land to build an orphanage. They hope to have more children of their own and still seek to improve the lives of other children in Ethiopia.

After the speech at the World Marathon Majors luncheon, Wami grasps the obligatory oversize check, walks back to her table and attempts to sit down with it. Jelena Prokopcuka happens to be sitting directly across from her and suddenly expresses a fervent interest in her baked salmon.

2:26:13—

Jelena Prokopcuka sprints across the finish line, punches her arms to the sky and throws her head back with a wide grin. The two-time defending champion looks as if she has just won the race.

"I'm very happy today, because I won the third place," she says to begin her press conference.

Some professional athletes scoff at moral victories, but although Prokopcuka neither crosses the finish line first nor collects the mother lode (she wins a modest $55,000), she believes in her accomplishment. She has still made the podium, having overcome her injury to pass two champions. She runs the only negative split of the top women, finishing the second half of the race in 1:12:50.

In three years, Prokopcuka has run six marathons and she has finished first twice, second twice and now third. She will win Latvian Sportswoman of the Year for the third consecutive time. Not a bad career so far, she reasons.

Radcliffe would be furious with third place. Actually, Radcliffe has never come in third place in a marathon.

"Paula is Paula," Prokopcuka and her husband will say, repeating their favorite mantra a couple more times over the next twenty-four hours.

Prokopcuka is comfortable with herself and her own values. She says that if or when she has a baby, she would likely take more time to recover before jumping back into training as Radcliffe did. "I care about myself, my husband," Prokopcuka says. "We have a different mental point of view, I have different limits, different threshold. Some people need the pain."

Prokopcuka was saddened by Ryan Shay's death, especially coming soon after her father-in-law died of a heart attack. When asked if she would continue her career if she knew of any potential risk to her health, Prokopcuka shakes her head firmly.

"My answer would be no," she says. "I have so many people who love me, and I can't afford to risk myself. It's my credo in life not to touch something if the price is too high."

She grows quiet before adding, "Maybe that's why I have not so many results."

Prokopcuka goes on, continuing in a torrent of English she could not even begin to speak in 2005, when she first won here. "Paula has had serious injuries. She's ready to pay the price. I'm not ready to pay that price," she says. "For me, sports, my career, I love what I do. But the body has limits. We have to respect our body, too. It's not worth it to do more than our body can take.

"I don't know if it is wise or not, but these are my feelings. With my price, I was able to be the two-time New York City champion. It's not so expensive. Fortunately, I have had no serious injury in my career and maybe because I wasn't so aggressive.

"I'm happy. And to be happy doesn't mean to have something more.

"To be happy," she concludes with a knowing smile, "is when you have enough."

2:09:04—

Martin Lel crosses the finish line flashing a pearly smile and spontaneously drops to the ground to plant a kiss on the asphalt, a marathon tradition. His body is fully extended, as if in a push-up. "I kissed the ground," he will say, "because I'd done good. It's wonderful."

Lel finishes 12 seconds in front of Abderrahim Goumri, having run an astonishingly fast negative split; he raced the second half of the Marathon in 1:03:19. And he ran the final 385 yards (sprinting the Marathon's point two) in 31 seconds.

Lel is overjoyed, running directly to hug his agent and his trainer who are off to the side of the finish line.

In only six weeks, however, Lel's elation will devolve into fear and sadness when he returns to Kenya. Violence erupts between rival tribes after the disputed election results of the country's president, Mwai Kibaki, on December 27. Lel's small grocery store still stands and his immediate family members living near Eldoret are safe, although more than one thousand people will die in wide-spread acts of violence between the Kalenjin tribe (to which Lel belongs) and the Kikuyu. Lucas Sang, a relay runner for Kenya at the 1988 Olympics, will be caught up in the fighting and macheted to death.

Lel stays close to his house and keeps a low profile. By the time he has recovered from New York, he will not be able to train long distances in the weeks after Christmas, since the outlying roads are blockaded. He tries to go to Uganda for a competition, "because I have pride in my country," he says, and is stranded at two local airports, returning after a treacherous day of ducking the street fighting.

He will go to a competition in Italy and then return to Kenya to check on his family before escaping the unrest to train in neighboring Namibia. Despite the disruption, in April 2008 Lel will win his third straight big-city marathon title, in London. Once again, he will outkick his competition to the finish line. He will pass Goumri, who will finish third behind Kenyan Sammy Wanjiru.

That fateful day in 2005 when an injured Lel watched from the New York Marathon stands as fellow Kenyan Paul Tergat out-sprinted Hendrick Ramaala to the tape gave Lel his motivation. "When you are hungry, it is not a problem," Lel would say about his uncanny finishing strength. "I am trained for this. In my mind I am going to fight to the finish."

2:09:16—

For the second major-city marathon in his career, Abderrahim Goumri finishes second to Lel. And yet the good-natured Moroccan seems content. He has won $65,000 for second place, plus a time bonus of $30,000.

"I come to New York to win the race—I did everything I could," Goumri says, although upon further reflection, he adds: "Next time I will not make the mistake to stay with Lel. He is so fast in the end."

Next time, it will be easier for Goumri to come to New York, because his U.S. visa lasts for three years. After the two weeks of visa anxiety that had followed four weeks of fasting for Ramadan, Goumri thinks these trials helped him.

"It is only the second big competition for me. I have to give thanks for God, I did a great race," he says.

2:11:25—
Hendrick Ramaala easily holds on to third place and qualifies for South Africa's Olympic team by 35 seconds.

"I did my job," he says after walking around the finish line with the South African flag. Ramaala grabs the last public time bonus that will be handed out today—$5,000—plus $40,000 for finishing third. He has now finished first, second and third in New York, and he is content with the race he ran today. Could Ramaala have won this race if he had not expended precious energy sprinting along stretches of Brooklyn or First Avenue? Probably not, considering Lel still has the best finishing kick in the business.

On First Avenue, Ramaala simply did what he has done every year he was in contention. Run that stretch with wild abandon. Later, Ramaala will hear from rival agents who were displeased with his tactics, mostly because he exhausted some runners who might have been in line for time bonuses had they run more conservatively.

"Do you think I care?" Ramaala says with a laugh. To those agents, whom he will not name, he says bluntly: "Next time teach your runners how to race."

The day after the Marathon, Ramaala will walk anonymously from his hotel down Seventh Avenue to the Toys "R" Us in Times Square—a sickly fluorescent three-story colossus with an indoor Ferris wheel and thousands of people, big and small, swarming the aisles. This is the one place in New York City that might be harder to navigate than all 26.2 miles of the Marathon, and certainly not at the pace of exactly 5 minutes per mile that Ramaala managed Sunday.

Making his way through the rows of action figures at his more comfortable, deliberate pace, Ramaala finds the kids' boxing gloves his son, Alex, has been begging for recently. Ramaala cannot come home from a business trip empty-handed.

He also must purchase a gift for Rodica; he tossed away his wife's favorite wool hat in Brooklyn when he grew too warm. He will have to replace it.

At the end of January, when South Africa turns to summer, he and Rodica celebrate the birth of their second child, a daughter they name Sarah Ioana, after Ramaala's mother and Rodica's father. Ramaala will sleep even less now. But as the seasons change and in April 2008 he adds a disappointing tenth-place finish in London to his résumé of twenty-two marathons, Ramaala will never stop running. It is his way.

2:46:43—

Lance Armstrong receives a champion's welcome at the finish line from Mayor Michael Bloomberg, who personally places the medal around Armstrong's neck. This time, Armstrong can smile without gritting his teeth. He ran 13 minutes faster this year than in his debut, giving him an average pace of 6 minutes, 21 seconds per mile.

Armstrong seems torn by his ferocious competitive spirit that compels him to beat the clock and his retired athlete persona that no longer wants to be restrained by time. "I've done a lot of things in my life fast, so it's now time to do them just for fun and recreation," he says.

In April 2008, he will run the Boston Marathon in 2:50:58.

3:47:19—

Pam Rickard has an added incentive on the way to the finish line.

Just as she enters the park at the Engineers' Gate, she encounters her only bit of New York hostility when a man behind her breaks the understood runners' code of conduct. He rudely pushes her, shouting: "Either move or get out of the way!"

Pam shouts back to him: "Hey, be nice!"

Pam is running with another woman, and they exchange exasperated looks in solidarity. Pam passes the man a half mile before the end.

It is not until she crosses that line that Pam sheds her first tears of the day, releasing the emotion she has controlled for the last 26.2 miles. She felt both the thrill and the sadness from having fulfilled her goal. Now what will she do?

After Pam ducks to collect her medal from the volunteer, she stops at the photography station and communicates in sign language to her husband: "I Love You." She gratefully accepts one of the foil mylar blankets that retain the heat and turn runners into plodding baked potatoes. She stops to lean her shoe on a wooden post to get her timing chip cut off by a seated volunteer, and then walks back into the sea of mylar, slipping upstream a quarter mile toward the UPS trucks to collect her baggage. It is chaotic again, and volunteers are sternly directing runners to keep moving. Pam obeys.

She finds the Central Park exit and anxiously goes to find her husband, Tom, on Central Park West.

"I qualified for Boston. I'm not going to do it, but I'm so grateful," Pam says, holding on to her husband.

"We'll see," Tom says with a smile.

Since Pam does not wear a watch, she does not realize that she has run faster than the 3:49 that flashed on the timer when she crossed the finish line. She does not know this until the week following the Marathon, when the New York Road Runners notifies her and 2,800 other runners in the orange corral that they have had a problem with the timing chips. The organizers ask runners to go by the honor system, to send in the times displayed on their watches. For those like Pam who were not wearing a watch or did not respond to an e-mail, the Road Runners subtracted three minutes from their recorded times since that is the elapsed time of the glitch their system determined.

According to Tom Kelley, the race-scoring director, a phone cable that ran under the timing mats for the orange start was somehow connected to the blue start for data communications, affecting the synchronization for the orange start. In other words: Their wires got crossed.

Either way, Pam qualifies for the Boston Marathon in April 2008. She checks herself and her ambition, trying to be satisfied with the high of what she just accomplished.

"I don't want to put you guys through that," she says to her husband. "Especially when I have to meet the group for 5:30 runs."

She knows it has not been easy for Tom to wake up before dawn to drive her there, go back to sleep and then pick her up. She gives him a big kiss and says, "That has been above and beyond the coaching duties."

She and Tom, instead, will go to Virginia Beach on March 16, 2008, where Pam will run the marathon and Tom will run the half-marathon. They will train together in the early mornings.

Pam will run 3:48:35, despite suffering a nasty bout of the flu for three weeks prior to the race. The Virginia Beach Marathon, in a sense, will seem almost "too normal," she will report. "No lottery, no four-plus-hour wait at Fort Wadsworth, no eavesdropping on animated conversations in other languages, no cannon, no people shamelessly peeing off a bridge, no five boroughs, no Olympic trials, no super-elites, no crowds that almost scare you with their cheering, no Stanley Rygor, no Central Park, and, they only hand you your medal, no put it around your sweaty, deserving neck!"

The New York City Marathon—Pam realizes—makes you feel like a superstar.

Even before her sobriety, Pam felt suited to the marathon because it was the one place where she could control herself. "I'd much rather master the distance than the speed," she said.

Only now, Pam understands she no longer needs a quick fix elsewhere in her life. In her quest to stay sober, she would always have a goal and a challenge in front of her.

"I am unspeakably proud of my Mom," Abby will say after the Marathon. "I could have never imagined the awesome person she has become or the incredible and so-much-more-than-restored relationship we've been blessed with."

When Pam returns from New York, she will place her medal around her four-year-old's neck, and Sophie will not take it off for a day and a half.

4:52:47—

Ellen and Larry Bakst sit in the stands at the finish line, Ellen's camera poised for the moment her sons have planned for months. Harrie and Rich cross the finish line holding hands and punching them to the sky.

"I was going to be there with you to cross the finish line, no matter what marathon hell you were going through," Rich says, standing with Harrie and his parents in the family reunion area on Central Park West. "It's the same way I was not going to let anyone else walk into the operating room with you. And God forbid, whatever happens or will happen, I will always be there."

Harrie is too overwhelmed with emotion and fatigue to make a similar speech. He just smiles and gives his brother a hug.

Later that evening, the Bakst family heads to the Crowne Plaza Hotel in Times Square for the Fred's Team reception. Harrie hears his name being called and sees people around him getting out of their chairs. Rich has to lift his brother out of his seat to acknowledge the standing ovation from more than 700 people.

"I still don't think Harrie realizes what he has done," Rich will say a day later.

That Monday morning, the brothers wear their medals and join members of Fred's Team for a visit to the pediatric cancer ward at Memorial Sloan-Kettering. The runners take pictures with the children, showing them their prizes, and visit the sicker patients in their rooms. It is both sobering and uplifting but a little distant to Harrie. He finds his connection later when he walks to the other end of the hospital he knows too well. Harrie visits his radiation therapist, Claire Markham, to share the experience of his race.

In April 2008, Rich will spend much more time on this floor. He would be accepted as a resident in Sloan-Kettering's radiation oncology department, one year and a week from the date Harrie started his radiation.

Even as they finish today's race, Harrie and Rich are planning for next year's New York City Marathon. And then, perhaps the Antarctica Marathon in 2009. Rich will get a late entry through Fred's Team to run the Boston Marathon in April. Harrie will be there to watch.

When Harrie goes home to his apartment after an unforgettable

Marathon Sunday, he flops on the couch in his living room, next to which sits his vase of dried eucalyptus leaves. They emit a faint aroma and radiate with meaning.

Harrie was inspired to buy them in late September after listening to a Yom Kippur sermon from his rabbi, Avi Weiss, a renowned Orthodox rabbi in the Bronx. Right before the traditional Yizkor memorial worship service, Rabbi Weiss preached about his favorite Israeli folk song, "The Eucalyptus Grove," by Israel's late national songwriter and poet, Naomi Shemer.

Shemer wrote the song in 1963 (twenty-two years before Harrie was born) to reflect the enduring power of the eucalyptus grove on the banks of the Jordan River. Her words depict the simple beauty of "the grove, the bridge, the boat, the fragrance of saltbush on the water" and how that scene will stay the same despite changes brought about by time, war, love and loss.

"We should be blessed to be blessed," Rabbi Weiss told his congregation that Yom Kippur day.

Harrie takes multiple meanings from the rabbi's message: He is grateful to be alive, while feeling blessed to realize the blessing of life itself. The eucalyptus leaves remind him daily of the unexpected difficulties and triumphs of his past year. He thinks of the sermon and how it reinforces his own motto: "Not to focus on what was lost, but to find value in what we have."

Harrie has a New York City Marathon medal and even better, five weeks later, he will have a clean cancer screen. His business will expand as he negotiates philanthropic opportunities for Soccer for Peace and enters into project discussions with the NBA.

Often, Harrie cannot believe what he has accomplished before the age of twenty-four. He tries not to think of an uncertain future, only knowing he is healthy now and that his family will always support him as they have during the past year.

"They were my eucalyptus grove," he says, "the constant through all of this, no matter what happened."

5:04:27—

Tucker Andersen and Joseph Shaw cross the finish line together. This is not Andersen's slowest marathon; he finished in 5:29 in 1985, the year he had cracked ribs. But this is a memorable one thanks to his television interview, conducted by the editor of *Runner's World*, David Willey.

"That will go in my tape library," Andersen says, dating himself with the technological reference.

Like other marathoners, Andersen does not mind the attention. There must be some payoff for getting up every day and not missing a day of running. He will fend off the flu later in the winter with the comfort of his routine and look forward to the Marathon in 2008.

5:29:58—

Here's the thing about celebrities in this city: True New Yorkers will act cool, noticing them but taking pains to leave them alone. Other times, New Yorkers are simply too busy to bother. The Marathon only intensifies this phenomenon.

Katie Holmes's handlers made sure that the New York Road Runners would not publicize her racing and that she could run the course in virtual anonymity; only a couple of tabloid Web sites picked up on her plan to run the Marathon. And yet, television cameras, magazine photographers and the New York tabloids are waiting for her at the finish line.

But where is Holmes?

Tom Cruise, Katie Holmes's megastar husband, has been waiting at the finish line for more than thirty minutes. Cruise holds the couple's daughter, Suri, on his shoulder and rocks her back and forth. He emerged from the VIP waiting room at Tavern on the Green early so that he would not miss his wife. He speaks to Road Runners chief, Mary Wittenberg, and conveys his wish to shield Holmes from the media, but he is also firm that she should finish the same way everyone else does. Meanwhile, runners pass Cruise, his hair still cut in character for the Nazi-era film he was shooting, and barely notice him. They are too wrapped up in their own drama.

Finally, there is excitement among the camera-wielding press who jostle for position when they hear she is approaching. Problem is—another celebrity is coming first. Just as the Road Runners officials are making sure that Holmes will be able to cross the line unencumbered by media, there comes Elton, aka Alexander Duszat. He is a portly 36-year-old German late-night television comedian who is the assistant to the lead host. And television crews have flown from Germany to record this moment.

Elton finishes his first marathon with a big, good-natured grin for the cameras. He looks around in amazement and exclaims to the German press: *"Dass war nicht normal!"*

Literally, that translates to: "That was not normal." The idiom means something along the lines of: "That was wicked."

His net time, from when he crossed the start line, will read 5:30:01. In real time that is about eight minutes before Holmes makes her way up the final hill. By the time the German reporters have cleared the finish line area, the rest of the cameras are ready. When she finally arrives in the far lane with her trainers doubling as bodyguards, she wears an FDNY baseball cap slightly askew, a spaghetti-strapped tank top, zip-up jacket and clingy sweatpants.

Suddenly, a loud cheer erupts from the stands.

The cheer is not for Holmes.

The fans are applauding Bill Reilly, a 55-year-old Brooklyn man with severe cerebral palsy, who is finishing at the same time. He has competed for twelve years in a row, all backward in his wheelchair. He kicks his feet to power his chair since he cannot use his legs. Reilly starts at 8 a.m. and finishes 7 hours, 50 minutes and 34 seconds later—a few feet away from Holmes. A member of the Achilles Track Club, Reilly is a fixture during weekend training sessions in Central Park and has quite a following.

When Cruise spots his wife he slips inside the finish line area, as arranged. He is there to place the medal around her neck. No ordinary Road Runners volunteer will do.

Holmes's entourage has suddenly grown, as six security people swarm the couple. For the first 18 miles of the race, she had her personal security at each mile's aid station, ready to sweep her away if she were injured or bothered. According to Road Runners, Holmes runs the entire Marathon at 12:37 per mile. It takes her 1 hour, 6 minutes to run the last four miles.

Holmes accepts congratulations from her family, and soon her security team whisks them into a waiting vehicle. She has a red carpet function to attend in New York that evening, to which she somehow wears high heels.

6:14:28—

Cindy Peterson holds hands with her three marathon buddies, Elyse Burden, Susan Rosmarin, and Linda Weissman, as they cross the finish line. They had a remarkably good time for running a marathon.

Cindy feels energized by walking every other mile. "I feel fabulous," she says. "There were people who were younger who were behind me.

"Every other marathon, by the time I get to the finish line, I'm almost in tears because I've run too much and I don't give myself breaks," she says. "I could do this again in another marathon and be better trained and run a faster time because I've been better rested."

She decides that it is worth it to have such an experience. "I made my PR in my hometown of Montreal, Canada, that was 4:45, and that was 1996. I'm not looking to make any records right now. I just want to be able to still run."

Now she has grand plans to check more off her list. Completing marathons in all continents and all fifty U.S. states is a common compulsion for some distance runners who consider the finish line a true destination.

"I want to finish my two continents," Cindy says. "And then my fifty states and make vacations around it. By then I'll be retired, over 70. I'm just very, very happy I'll be able to do this."

The afternoon light is fading into dusk. Central Park's West Drive is littered with bagels, banana peels, cups, plastic bottles, gloves, sweat bands, energy-bar wrappers—the debris of a day's work. It will take a week before the West Drive opens to traffic again. Cindy arrives at her designated UPS truck to get her baggage, only there is commotion and uproar at the truck designated for late finishers. It seems that the overwhelmed workers cannot find the bags for some runners, many of whom are over 50 years old and must sit down on the curb, shivering and exhausted. Runners are shouting and pushing, and Cindy manages to escape after waiting only fifteen minutes.

Earlier, in the hour when the majority of finishers crossed the line—4:28:38 is the median time—the road became overcrowded with runners wrapped in mylar, all walking north (some more than a half mile) to pick up their clear plastic bags of clothing from the UPS trucks. There was so little space that people were elbowing for room, yelling impatiently and complaining loudly.

And with that, New York's marathon bubble bursts. For one magnificent morning and afternoon, participants get to run in suspended reality. They enter a glorified theme park—"New York, New York!"—where roads are closed just for them, people hand them water, bunting hangs on city fences, bands are playing, choirs are harmonizing, people are cheering and holding signs, and everyone is getting along.

But eventually, the chill sets in, the fantasy fades along with the sun and the real New York slowly creaks back to life. Suddenly people remember they are in pain. They are cold and cranky and just want to figure out how to get back to their hotels or apartments or cars. No bands are saluting people now. They are on their own—at least until the Marathon-sponsored dance party later that night.

As Cindy heads out of the park and onto Central Park West, where runners are supposed to reunite with friends and families, she looks at Salazar's inscription on the back of her medal. She agrees that the triumph of the will "above all limits" includes age limits. "I'm glad he said that, because it's so true," Cindy says.

She puts on some warm layers and starts searching for her boyfriend, Ron. Ten minutes and a few cell phone snafus later, they see each other on the street corner and Ron gives her a big kiss.

"I love this gal," he says. "She's a very special lady. No matter what she does, she succeeds at it. Singer, a DJ, dancer, runner, her job, a lover, what can I tell you?"

Please, Ron, not more than that.

The two laugh. Cindy is radiant beneath her sparkling red and purple cap, her two-carat diamond earrings flashing in the street lights of Central Park West. Her mascara and lipstick are still on, 14 hours later. It is time to take her makeup off.

A recorded announcement booms in a monotone over a six-language loop: "The finisher area is now closing. If you still have not reunited with your runner or your family, please come to the information booth on 72nd Street."

The Marathon officially ends 6 hours and 40 minutes from the time the cannons blast on the Verrazano-Narrows Bridge.

Monday morning, the fastest woman on two feet and the slowest woman on two feet will meet at the finish line for a photo op. Zoe Koplowitz, 59, crosses the line in front of the waiting cameras and in front of Paula Radcliffe. Koplowitz, who has diabetes and multiple sclerosis, completes her twentieth New York City Marathon in 27 hours and 45 minutes. She has help from her annual Hell's Angels escort through Upper Manhattan and the Bronx in the middle of the night to become the last—though unofficial— finisher.

The runners who finished in less than 5 hours will be listed in the results page of the *New York Times*' special Monday Marathon section. At Tavern on the Green, a line snakes around the corner, as many runners read the paper in the queue while waiting to have their medals engraved with their name and times.

Many will experience the inevitable marathon letdown, the withdrawal from having trained so long for a one-day event. But for a few more hours Monday, the resplendent sunbeams allow for a little more basking.

New York becomes the world's largest medal stand as people preen around the city, or in airports, showing off their prize. It is the key to an exclusive club, an instant status symbol, license to walk slowly, eat plentifully, gloat, groan and grin.

The medal is an invitation to tell a story.

ACKNOWLEDGMENTS

Life, as the saying goes, is a marathon. Thank goodness for that. I am not a fan of sprints.

The marathon is indeed an apt metaphor for all we do. The 26.2-mile race demands discipline, perseverance and luck. It rewards the crazy, but still celebrates the plodder. Of all the sports that I have covered in my seventeen-year journalism career—from Olympic track and field to professional basketball, high school football to professional tennis—no event more than the Marathon best captures the whole of the human experience. Or, for that matter, the book-writing experience.

The similarities struck me at every turn. I prepared diligently, stretched my limits and experienced the writer's high. I also hit The Wall. I managed to reach the finish line, again and again. And I never would have made it were it not for my good friends, family and colleagues.

To produce an event that truly is like no other race in the world, the New York Road Runners takes one full year to organize. Add another high-profile marathon to the weekend—the United States Olympic men's marathon trials—and the enormity of the task becomes overwhelming. The Road Runners pulled it off on the weekend of November 3 and 4, thanks to a passionate staff, plus an enthusiastic volunteer corps of thousands. I am extremely grateful for the support and the access the Road Runners gave me in writing this book, which they endorsed from the start but never tried to restrict.

I first must thank Mary Wittenberg, the chief executive officer of the New York Road Runners, for believing in this project—and in me—from the beginning. I marvel at her indefatigable spirit and her optimism. I appreciate her compassion, her friendship and her time—all those weekend hours after races that she spent with me instead of her loving family, her husband, Derek, and sons Alex and Cary.

The Road Runners' media relations director, Richard Finn, whom I have known since we covered the United States Open, first discussed the concept with me and I ran with it at the right time. My thanks extend to everyone at the Road Runners, and to the inner circle, who graciously answered my frequent requests: Sam Grotewold, David Monti, Sara Hunninghake, Susan Cuttler, Peter Ciaccia, Tom Kelley, Ann Hinegardner, Bob Laufer, Gordon Bakoulis, Richard Hulnick, Steve Boland, Pat McNamara, David Katz, Jillian Haber, Ian Brooks, Alice Yoo, Stephanie Ross and Arnold Sitruk. I am thankful for the archives coming from the minds and homes of George Hirsch, the chairman of the board of the Road Runners, and Allan Steinfeld, the former chief executive and president of the Road Runners, who loves the Marathon as much as his friend Fred Lebow did, and is still an ambassador for the sport.

I cherish the encouragement as well as the recollections Grete Waitz offered me throughout this project. Grete is a champion in her own class, a woman so gracious and so grounded, she has touched us all with her strength.

This book would not have words were it not for three very important friends who edited tirelessly and helped me get past many Walls. Lori Shontz and I became lifetime friends after closing down the press room at the 1996 Atlanta Olympics' final competition while writing the inspiring story of South Africa's Josia Thugwane winning the men's marathon. From wire to wire, including Marathon weekend in New York, Lori kept me sane and focused with her insightful editing and reassurance—even while uprooting her life to become the weekend sports editor at the *Miami Herald*. Her 2001 Pew Fellowship project on women runners in Kenya, published in the Pittsburgh *Post Gazette*, guided me throughout my own experience.

Carl Nelson, the incomparable *New York Times* night sports editor, approached every word with tremendous generosity, honesty and patience. He provided his nonrunner's perspective and picked up the phone at all hours of the night to offer encouragement. Peter Krebs, a visionary artist and an invaluable, do-everything member of the Road Runners family, enabled me to see new ways to tell this story in words and pictures. Ballygally.

Joe Drape, my esteemed *Times* colleague, convinced me to write my first book, connected me with my agent, Andrew Blauner, and he reminded me to relax. Neil Amdur, the sports editor who hired me nine years ago, is a marathon aficionado; his decades of reporting for the *Times*—notably his coverage of Rosie Ruiz's saga—gave me a brilliant model of how to "nail" a story. I frequently consulted Jere Longman's beautifully written running pieces from the *Times*. I am grateful to Fern Turkowitz, for helping me transition to my book leave, and to Craig Hunter for his technical and emotional support.

Maria Farnon, my longest running friend, offered such detailed notes from the men's press truck and from the finish line on race day that I referred to them every day in the writing process. Jane Shapiro shared her triumphant first-timer's experience and always lent an ear. Thanks to: Larry Freed for being there; Toby Tanser, for his expert knowledge of Kenya and the New York running scene; Barbara Charles, for connecting me with her teammates on the Mercury Masters; Susan Cosier, for research; Marty Post, for his statistical analysis of Paula Radcliffe's and Gete Wami's rivalry. Ryan Lamppa, of Running USA, for 2007 figures. Dr. Dave Martin, for knowing everything about the marathon and for providing a physical breakdown of the race's effects. Jimmy Lynch, who helped me overcome my own physical breakdowns and start running for real. And Debra Gill, for helping me tap into runners' psyches and my own.

I thank two first-timers I met while chatting about the book in restaurants: Steve Gonzales offered unbridled excitement and observation, as did Albert Belman.

Since the marathon is a journey of discovery, I could not have done without Janet Sporleader at Anthony Travel; she rescued me and got me seamlessly to South Africa and back. In Johannesburg, Rodica Moroianu and Hendrick Ramaala opened their home and their life to me. Thanks to Rodica for her carrot soup, muffins, cookies and porridge. I am grateful to Craig Cynkin, a runner in Ramaala's group, and to his parents, Neville and Gillian, for welcoming me into their *sukkah*. Thanks to Jelena Prokopcuka and her husband, Aleks, for showing me around Jurmala, and for Jerry Wirth's expert tour in Riga. I was happy for the hospitality in London from good friend Jennifer Quinn, and Jim Watkins. In California, Cheryl Rosenberg Neubert blogged her support.

Closer to home, I can't think of anybody better suited to be my editor than Kate Hamill, a 3-hour marathoner who has run New York three times and embraced this idea from the start. Her unwavering belief in the power of the New York City Marathon informed my writing, making this by far a better book. As for my agent, Andrew, from our common love of all things Peanuts, we always saw the book from the same perspective—embracing the wit, the pathos and the dizzying possibility of the First Sunday in November.

And finally, at the end of this marathon of thanks, I extend my love and gratitude to my family. To my cousins Rabbi Dan Fink, who reviewed my chapter on Fred Lebow and the Williamsburg Hasidim; Julie Fink, who helped me with Virginia court records; Jon and Betty Fink, San Antonio Spurs fans, who supported my previous NBA-writing career; my cousin Betsy Hirsch, who ran New York four times, and who, along with her friend Lynn Canfield, gave me their volunteer perspectives; my aunts, Karen Fink, who has always showered me with love, and Judy Robbins, who has always known me so well and given me Zen-like guidance. My late uncle Marty, her husband, is the reason why I am an author today. I reread his books of poetry for inspiration, remembering when I was four years old how we used to compose stories on the typewriter together.

And last, but really first, I must thank my parents, Wendy and Larry, both published authors in their own right. You welcomed me to the club and reminded me, with love, to bend my knees to achieve what I have today.

SELECTED BIBLIOGRAPHY

Amdur, Neil. "New Doubts on Woman Runner Who Won Marathon Are Raised." *New York Times*, April 23, 1980.

Broadbent, Rick. "Paula Radcliffe Fears Another Olympic Failure." *Times* (London), May 10, 2008, http://www.timesonline.co.uk/tol/sport/olympics/article3904707.ece.

Eskanazi, Gerald. "In This Marathon They Also Run Who Only Sit and Wait." *New York Times*, October 2, 1972.

Fixx, James F. *The Complete Book of Running*. New York: Random House, 1977.

Kolata, Gina. "Training Through Pregnancy to Be Marathon's Fastest Mom." *New York Times*, November 3, 2007.

Kuscsik, Nina. "Marathon: More Than a Mania; Veteran Looks Back and Ahead." *New York Times*, October 25, 1981.

Lebow, Fred, with Richard Woodley. *Inside the World of Big-Time Marathoning*. New York: Rawson Associates, 1984.

Longman, Jere. "In Ethiopia, Mercury Soaring." *New York Times*, February 1, 2007.

Martin, David E., and Roger W. H. Gynn. *The Olympic Marathon. The History and Drama of Sports' Most Challenging Event*. Champaign, Illinois: Human Kinetics, 2000.

McKinley, James C., Jr. "Wheelchair Racers Seek Equality with Runners." *New York Times*, November 4, 1999.

Meili, Trisha. *I Am the Central Park Jogger: A Story of Hope and Possibility*. New York: Scribner, 2003.

Radcliffe, Paula, with David Walsh. *Paula: My Story So Far*. London: Simon & Schuster, 2004.

Rastorfer, Darl. *Six Bridges: The Legacy of Othmar H. Ammann*. New Haven, Connecticut: Yale University Press, 2000.

Selected Bibliography

Redelmeir, Donald A., and J. A. Greenwald. "Competing Risks of Mortality with Marathons: Retrospective Analysis." *British Journal of Medicine*, December 22, 2007, http://www.bmj.com/cgi/content/full/335/7633/1275.

Roberts, William O., and Barry J. Maron. "Evidence for Decreasing Occurrence of Sudden Cardiac Death Associated with the Marathon." *Journal of the American College of Cardiology*, October 2005; 46:1373–1374 (published online 15 September 2005). http://content.onlinejacc.org/cgi/content/full/46/7/1373.

Rubin, Ron. *Anything for a T-Shirt: Fred Lebow and the New York City Marathon, the World's Greatest Footrace.* Syracuse: Syracuse University Press, 2004.

Switzer, Kathrine. *Marathon Woman: Running the Race to Revolutionize Women's Sports.* New York: Carroll and Graf, 2007.

Switzer, Kathrine, and Roger Robinson. *26.2 Marathon Stories.* Toronto: Madison Press Books, 2006.

Talese, Gay. *The Bridge.* New York: Harper & Row, 1964.

Tanser, Toby. *The Essential Guide to Running the New York City Marathon.* New York: Berkley Publishing Group, 2003.

Thigpen, David E. "Meltdown: What Really Happened in Chicago." *Runners World*, February 2008.

Vecsey, George. "New York City Marathon: Fred and Grete Win All of New York City." *New York Times*, November 2, 1992.

Vecsey, George. "New York City Marathon: In All the Boroughs, the Crowds Came Out to Honor Lebow." *New York Times*, November 7, 1994.

Waitz, Grete, with Gloria Averbuch. *Run Your First Marathon: Everything You Need to Know to Reach the Finish Line.* New York: Skyhorse Publishing, 2007.

INDEX

Index

Lough, Isla, 18–19, 79, 161, 162, 294, 296–97

Lucky Dube, 50

Madison Avenue Bridge, 232

Madsen, Marissa, 30

Maffei, Louis, 90–91

Maharam, Lewis, 265, 267

Maimonides, Moses, 112

Malcolm X, 232

Malone, Clint, 271–75

Malone, Jackson, 273–74

Malone, Jennifer, 271–75

Manhattan, 169–71, 181–82, 200

Manhattan Avenue, Brooklyn, 133–37

Manhattan Furrier, 136

Marathon Blue (color), 166–68

Marathon Expo, 17

marathons, 6, 25
  deaths and, 268
  length of, 6, 20, 287
  spirituality and, 15–16, 55–57
  training for, 84, 101, 102, 103, 143, 160–61, 257, 263, 264, 267–68
  women and, 208–12
  See also specific marathons

Marcus Garvey Park, 237

Marine Corps Marathon, 3, 28

Markham, Claire, 171–72, 175, 307

Martin, Dave, 219, 220, 267

Mary Gladys, Sister, 130

Masilela, Isaac, 54

Mayor's Cup, 33

McCabe, Charlie, 234

McCarren Park, Brooklyn, 133

McGrory, Amanda, 123, 125–26, 131

McReilly's Pub, 149

Meili, Trish, 254–55

Memorial-Sloan Kettering Cancer Center, 12, 171–72, 175, 177–78, 307

Mendelsohn, Steve, 149–50

Mercury Masters, 16, 93, 206, 207

Metropolitan Pool, 121

Mexico, 280–81

Monti, David, 53, 260

Moroianu, Rodica, 46, 185, 187–88, 190–92, 241, 303

Morrow, Susan, 287

Moses, Robert, 29

Moten, Billie, 197

motherhood, 19, 41, 79, 83, 85, 112, 159, 161

Moyo (restaurant), 186–87

Mtolo, Willie, 189

Muhrcke, Gary, 210

Index